AN EVER ROLLING STREAM

To Gillian
With lots of love from the author
June 2nd 2015

AN EVER ROLLING STREAM

FROM THE CONVENTIONAL TO THE
UNCONVENTIONAL IN LIFE
(AND MEDICINE)

DON SNUGGS

Copyright © 2015 Don Snuggs

The moral right of the author has been asserted.

Apart from any fair dealing for the purposes of research or private study, or criticism or review, as permitted under the Copyright, Designs and Patents Act 1988, this publication may only be reproduced, stored or transmitted, in any form or by any means, with the prior permission in writing of the publishers, or in the case of reprographic reproduction in accordance with the terms of licences issued by the Copyright Licensing Agency. Enquiries concerning reproduction outside those terms should be sent to the publishers.

Matador
9 Priory Business Park
Kibworth Beauchamp
Leicestershire LE8 0RX, UK
Tel: (+44) 116 279 2299
Fax: (+44) 116 279 2277
Email: books@troubador.co.uk
Web: www.troubador.co.uk/matador

ISBN 978-1784622-718

British Library Cataloguing in Publication Data.
A catalogue record for this book is available from the British Library.

Typeset in Aldine by Troubador Publishing Ltd
Printed and bound in the UK by TJ International, Padstow, Cornwall

Matador is an imprint of Troubador Publishing Ltd

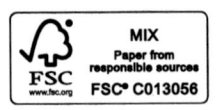

ALSO BY THE SAME AUTHOR

To Travel Hopefully
Twenty-two years in the RAF medical branch

Reuben the Fisherman
A tale of Roman occupied Palestine

Lydia's Dream
A Roman Lady who saw history made

CONTENTS

PART ONE	1

My Parents	3
Childhood Memories	8
Life at Westbury Infant School	12
The New World of the Grammar School	26
Life Gets Serious	38
The Real World	41
Getting to Grips with the Job	47
Postscript to Part One	53

PART TWO	57

Prologue	59
New Beginnings	61
Under New Leadership	67
Waking Up	78
A Student Again	84
Traditional Chinese Medicine	89
Interlude	96
Building a Practice	101
The Learning Curve Steepens	114
Life Gets Serious	125
Thinking Outside the Box	130
Getting the Message Across	138
Helping the Lost!	148
Getting to Grips with Routine	156
Day to Day Problems	174
The Door Closes But Another Opens	179
Postscript	190

To the memory of my parents

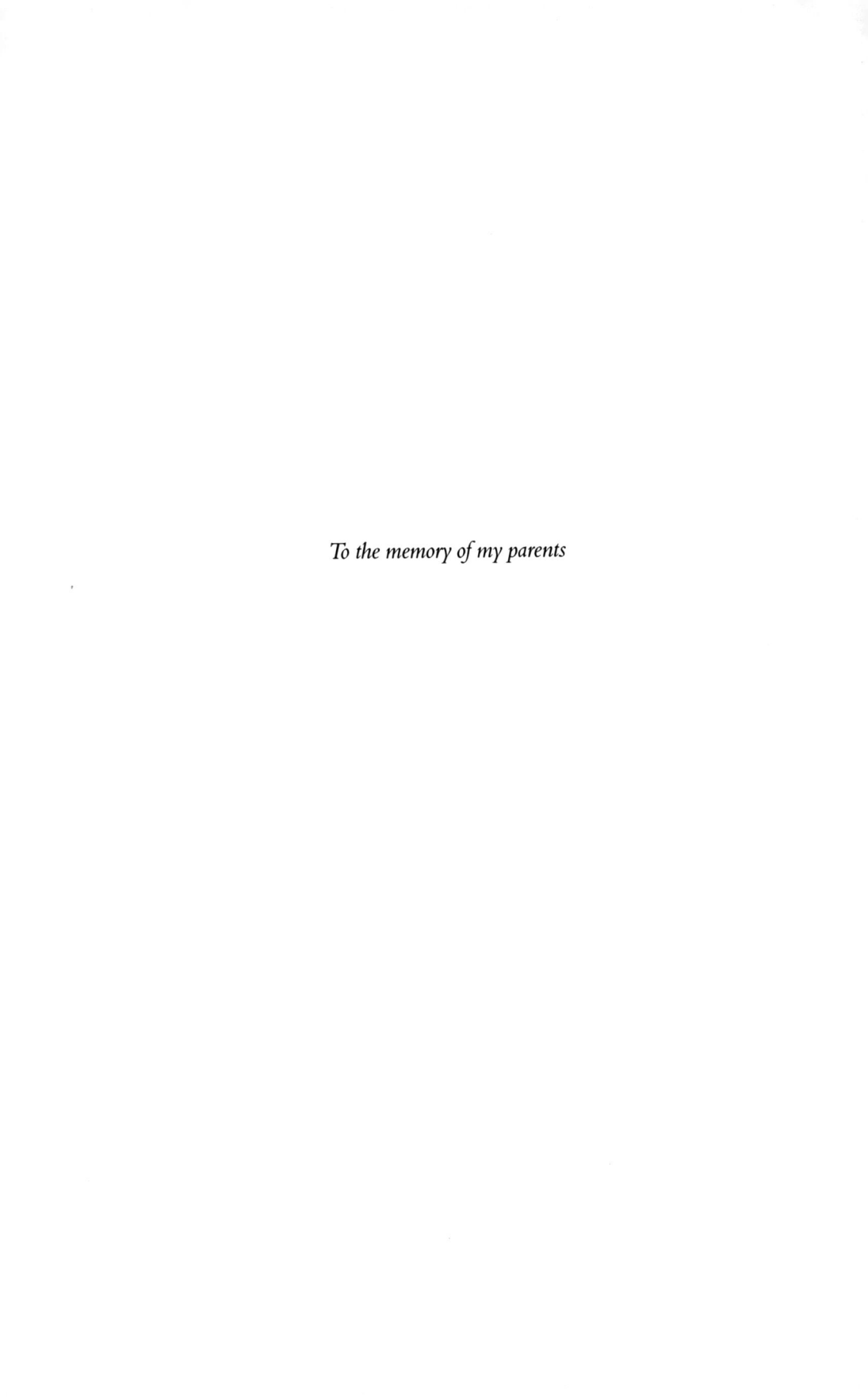

PART ONE

Time like an ever-rolling stream
bears all its sons away,
they fly forgotten as a dream
dies at the opening day.

Isaac Watts 1748

1

MY PARENTS

"What the policeman!" my father would explode when confronted with some inexplicable situation. This was the nearest that he, a very moral man, would ever come to using an expletive, and I have never before or since heard that phrase from any other person but himself, although in old age I occasionally use it myself, much to the amusement of my dear wife! It probably reflects in some measure the esteem in which that body of public servants were held at that time, compared with the attitude of the general public and media today. But from my father, never was a profanity allowed to cross his lips. His culture was always one in which good manners and exemplary behavior were the order of the day, and respect for his betters, irrespective of any situation in which he found himself.

He was a product of his time. The eldest son of a big family, he was born in 1903. His father, a general dealer and a pillar of the local Strict Baptist chapel whose outward sign of piety, in a rather stratified society, was that of shabby gentility and absolute respectability. His business was in a small Bedfordshire village, which had changed little over the years in size or attitudes. Suits were worn on a Sunday, and for Sunday only, observations of the Sabbath were rigidly implemented and the uniform for this was the suit, usually with a bowler hat. There was within the clan, as it were, a sense that 'we are not like the others, we stand apart', unless of course there was a good deal to be done, and at that point they joined the club!

Grandfather was a very conservative man; his whole life was guided by his principles and by prayer. I recall only one major thing about him other than his bushy moustache, very common in those days, and that was his total mistrust of doctors, and that after a period of severe abdominal pain he was diagnosed with cancer of the bowel and was told that unless he was operated on immediately he would die; he replied to the senior surgeon, " Not before my time young man."

At the top of the heap in the village, of course, was the squire; he was a churchman, he had to be. The Church of England in those days was the 'Tory party at prayer' and although the squire stood above the rest, he was viewed with suspicion by the working and labouring classes. However, it was to this august man that everyone went in times of trouble, and indeed we are told voted as he suggested they should at elections, thus keeping in with this rather anachronistic relic of the Middle Ages was a wise move.

The middle classes were beginning to emerge from this hierarchical arrangement: the doctor who was now better educated than his forbears over the centuries, free from mysticism and witchcraft, and although he could rarely prescribe anything better that a white or red medicine, wrapped in a cream coloured paper and sealed with red sealing wax, he was recognised as a wise man who attempted to smooth the path of the sick on their downhill journey; the parson who was now influenced by the Oxford movement, and did his best to bring to the old miserable services of the church a bit of colour and awe to his rambling sermons; the solicitor, who with the rise of a more compassionate society of would-be benefactors in the later part of Victoria's reign, could to some extent understand the political and social turmoil which came with the end of the old queen's reign, and the changes in society that would soon follow, culminating in the dreadful bloodletting of the First World War, with all its misery and pain.

My father died when I was fifteen in 1947. I therefore had little knowledge of him as anything other than an authoritarian figure, but he was thought of by all as a very good man, and my memories of him were unlike those of somebody who would know his parents into old age. Thus my memories are those of a teenager; but I have gradually changed the opinion I had of him then, with my experiences of life and all the many changes that come with the developments in society. I now view his memory with some degree of sympathy for the many artificial restrictions placed upon him that his background deemed necessary in those far off times, although by and large, they, and people of his ilk, rested content within those same restrictive practices.

He was educated in the village school, had a good knowledge of mathematics which served him well, he was a natural mechanic, wrote with a well rounded hand, as most people of his generation had to, left school at fourteen, was apprenticed to a watchmaker, and towards the end of his comparatively short life, became a scientific instrument maker, at which trade he excelled. So he was very much a product of his upbringing with all its taboos and restrictions. He was not so far as I can recall a very demonstrative man, he was I believe a very just man, and inculcated in myself and my two brothers a great sense of justice, but he was not particularly aware of all that was happening in life, being a member of his church in which he held the post of deacon, which he felt separated him somewhat from those who held no faith at all. 'You don't want to have anything to do with that sort of thing' was often his advice, I'm sure he would have been appalled to think however that he consciously avoided contacts with others who did not share his beliefs and faith; it was a subconscious act brought about by his narrow upbringing as much as anything, and the times in which he lived, with limited communications apart from a battery radio of low range, and a newspaper which like any other even now gives the reader a slant on the news that is biased in favour of some faction. But it did not preclude him from having ambition for me and my two brothers, that we should get a job in an office. To him as a blue-collar worker, as it was known in those days, working in an office was the epitome of success, having little idea that there was a pecking order even in that!

He was hard working; he not only had a job in a shop in the town (he'd moved to Letchworth Garden City when he and Mother married in 1927), he had a small bench in the 'living room' as it was known, shielded from prying eyes by a wallpaper-covered screen which had a motif of blue flowers. The pattern always intrigued me as a child. Behind the screen he did private work, mending watches and clocks in what little time he had which was not taken up in church matters. This supplementary income in those recessionary times enabled us to live modestly, and allowed us a week by the sea once a year.

He was not a gardener, and just liked to keep the grass short at the front of the house so that it was tidy. The back, I recall, was left to fend for itself, and we kids did what we wanted in it without fear of retribution!

In his dress he was neat and tidy, shoes highly polished and shirt collars well starched, and always immaculately shaven. In fact looking back on him after all these years, he was the model respectable working man who knew his place in society and was proud of it! Some little while ago I found among some old family papers a reference given to him by his employer before he left the shop, directed as many were to war work in 1939 in the factories. It described him as a man of impeccable character, and I believe he was just that.

He was not, unfortunately, endued with a great sense of humour, probably knocked out of him by his upbringing; he didn't tell jokes and preferred not to listen to them, but would occasionally smile at some of the antics that came with ITMA and Tommy Handley, which for some reason we were allowed to listen to when the radio battery was charged up enough.

But Mother was of different material, she had an impish sense of laughter and would make some very funny comments at times which were usually most perceptive. I always recall her telling me in confidence – 'and don't tell your father', she said – that as a child on her first day at school, she heard a boy refer to his bottom as his bum. Unfortunately when she went home that evening she used this term, and for her pains was threatened that she would have her mouth washed out with soap and water if she said it again. However the word stuck in her mind and she could not get it out of her system, so one day in sheer frustration she went down to the riverside where it was very quiet, and with nobody around shouted the word at the top of her voice until she was exhausted!

Mother was also from the same background, but from a city. She was the youngest daughter in a family of eight children. Her father was a businessman who was also a lay preacher in the Strict Baptist circuit. Quite well-to-do, they lived in a large town house of some three stories high in Luton, in which I can remember as a small child getting lost!

Mother had much the same type of upbringing as my father, but she had worked after she left school in a big drapery store in London and lived over the shop. She was very musical, not an attribute in the opinion of her parents, but she had a lovely soprano voice which had she been allowed adequate training would have taken her to unimagined heights in the music circles of the day; but as a woman, and as a member of the Strict Baptist chapel, she was expected to show no signs of elitism (this would have been designated as pride by the faithful), but to know her place and become a good wife and mother, and indeed she became just that!

She was always neatly dressed, and pictures of her in her youth show her to be an attractive young lady, an acceptable catch for any young man from the same background. My parents met because of their family membership of the chapel circuit. They were married in 1927 at the chapel in Luton which is still there, and I am told has a fair membership. They always used their faith to guide them in all decisions in their lives, and rested content within the limitations it set on them; proscriptive it may have been as I look at it from some eighty years on, but it gave direction to their lives and they rested spiritually comfortable within its enveloping arms.

So these were the two ordinary, but rather wonderfully content and hard working people, who gave me my being, and I'm sure that their influence has been the cause of my well fulfilled existence, giving me direction 'in all the changing scenes of life in trouble and in joy' and I think from Mother in particular, a great sense of humour, and I revere their memory.

2

CHILDHOOD MEMORIES

My earliest memory of the town in which I was born was accompanying my mother on a shopping trip in my pram.

I recall quite vividly sitting up in my harness, facing the direction of travel and pretending to be a bus driver. I was intrigued with the big green buses of the Eastern National bus company which seemed to have the monopoly of public transport in that pre-war era, and I had perfected the art of mimicking bus engine noises, or so I thought! Each bus had a distinctive engine noise, and I could vary the sound according to the type of bus I wanted to be at the time, either a Bristol, or even a Dennis – this one was the most difficult because it had a whine on top of its usual diesel noise – or the very best, and there were not a lot of these, the Leyland! The quietest and smoothest of the lot, and as I was aware, it had six cylinders rather than the usual five in the others, which were to me, lesser makes!

I can remember ignoring the comments of those who spoke to my mother as she chatted with friends; we had after all stopped to pick up passengers, what else does a bus stop for? And the driver had enough to do controlling this huge 'double-decker' without indulging in small talk with a passer-by! When they had finished talking I rang the imaginary bell and we proceeded on our way to the sound of the appropriate engine noise.

My favourite part of the town was just outside the Midland Bank where there were always buses waiting to pick up their load; people getting on buses, and coming down the stairs from the upper deck, absolute controlled turmoil to a two-year-old, desperately wanting to go for a ride on the monster.

The town for me in those days was a huge place. Letchworth was actually a fairly small town and has not grown a lot to this day, but it was of course to us the centre of the universe, and to me, full of buses!

However, the time came when I was old enough to have my first bus journey to Luton to see some relatives, and to my disgust it turned out badly and I threw up all over the seats with motion sickness which lasted until I had my appendix out some years later. To everyone's surprise, and to my great relief, surgery cured me of this unpleasant affliction. Not a recommended remedy for the problem however!

I had an elder brother who was proving to be very clever and learning to play the piano; he was having lessons at an early age and it was expected, I was told later, that I would emulate his prowess and we would become a famous musical family in the town. I did like music, but as a strict chapel family, the type of music we were allowed to listen to was very limited. Jazz was anathema, swing most unacceptable, so it was classical or nothing.

Letchworth was a somewhat arty place with all kinds of odd people living there, it had been formed only forty or so years ago and attracted the artistic classes, but most of my day to day life was of course in the home, playing in the garden. We were taken to chapel on a Sunday morning, where I was forced to sit on wickerwork seats which irritated the backs of my legs. I could not understand what was going on, but loved the singing, unless my mother, who was a soprano and sang like a bird, occasionally lapsed into the contralto which did not please me, and I would stop singing and nudge her and tell her to stop. If I was too disruptive I recall being taken outside by Mother and given a smack on the bottom, taken back and told in no uncertain terms that there was more where that came from if I mucked about again in the service, and that the smack hurt her more than it hurt me! While she was performing this punishment on me, with a stinging bottom, I never could get my head round that one! But my life and that of my elder brother was full of love; Mother was a truly loving person and my father, for all his strict ways, was a comfortable man to be with when you learnt his funny ways.

I will always remember being in bed on a Sunday evening, when Mother and my brother were at the evening service, my father hammering out hymns inexpertly on the piano and singing to them in a not very tuneful voice. He played the piano using the old tonic-sol-fa notation, which limited him to only four part harmony, but it was comforting and part of my life, familiar and looked forward to in days before T.V. and before radio programmes were considered suitable or available for we children on a Sunday evening.

Sunday school on Sunday afternoon was obligatory of course. We would sit in circles listening to the 'teachers' reading us Bible stories and singing choruses; all of course had a very simple message in them, mainly about being good children, and if we were very good, we would one day all meet together in heaven!

Childhood illnesses were a constant threat to our survival before the war: diphtheria was the most dreaded, persons who contracted this disease were confined to the fever hospital for three months' quarantine and often suffered severe side effects if they survived, which caused all kinds of problems in later life; measles with its subsequent ear infections and sometimes mastoiditis which required surgery. In those days prior to antibiotics, children with chicken pox, with its very irritant skin rash which scabbed, couldn't leave these alone, and often ended up with secondary infected lesions which were unsightly. I still have, eighty-one years later, a recognisable scar on my arm from this. There was also a risk of meningitis following this disease; it was not uncommon to hear of families devastated by the loss of youngsters from these diseases which are now confined to the third world, hopefully, but war or famine, prejudice or social unrest, could cause them again to raise their ugly heads.

My first remembered holiday was to St Osyth in Essex. I was in the final state of chicken pox and still scratching but was deemed fit enough to travel, so long as I avoided contact with other children. We were to be transported by a senior member of the chapel for this week's delight; going in a car was excitement enough, and for my first visit to the seaside this added to the fun, but I did my usual thing and threw up all over the car before we were half way there!

We stayed in a small chalet on the sea bank. I can recall waking up the first morning looking out of the French doors to this blue sea; there before me was a Thames barge which had anchored a few yards from the beach, waiting for the tide to turn. Whenever I see such vessels on the T.V. programmes today, it takes me back to that wonderful morning; not only the sea, but a ship as well! What more could a lad want?

The accommodation was basic, but average for the times; there was no running water, just a standpipe at the end of the row of chalets. Toilet facilities were even more basic, and waste had to be emptied from the chamber pot each morning into a cesspit further along the shore, but this did not spoil the enjoyment of the week's break.

I still have a very grainy photograph of us all as a family walking along what could, with a bit of imagination, be called a promenade, all in our best clothes of course; just because we were on holiday didn't mean you went scruffily dressed, my father's only concession to relaxation was to wear canvas shoes and not to wear a tie! The picture was obviously taken by one of the seaside photographers, a common sight as they carried out their trade looking for willing customers. It was almost obligatory to go home with a group photo to show the folks at home that we had been away.

By this time the family had increased to three boys; my new brother was born when I was four years old. I can still remember how placid a child he was, but merited little of my attention initially as yet I couldn't play with him. But we were a happy little family, well contained in our own little world, loved by our parents and frequently visited by doting relatives. This happy state lasted until the prospect of school suddenly burst upon me, and another world was entered with all its terror and expectations.

3

LIFE AT WESTBURY INFANT SCHOOL

'Like a snail unwillingly to school'? Well it wasn't quite like that; Mother took me to the school one day to meet the head teacher. She was a matronly figure who rejoiced in the name of Miss Virgin, and after all the usual business of form filling I was allocated to the first primary class under the benevolent care of one Mrs Dear, who came from the same village that was the original home of my father.

I can recall with amusement only some of the goings on that day, the little girl called Jane who dirtied her knickers, Stanley who sat next to me who arrived with a thick coating of white sugar round his mouth from the sticky unwrapped doughnut which, with delight, he brought with him in his pocket! Neil who was in tears and wanted his mum, and so on. It was a group essentially from a working-class area, but there was one posh girl called Cynthia. I never did know why she was there because her parents were both doctors, but this disparate group settled down together and we learned to sing 'Three Green Bottles' and other such musical gems, the act of singing making us all feel better, and indeed that we belonged to class one infants.

It was on reflection, after we had found our feet, a happy group, but we were subjected to strong discipline; no really meant no, I had my bare leg slapped by the teacher for touching the piano in the hall, I couldn't see why, after all we had a piano at home and whenever I walked passed that I donged a note, but we had been told not to touch it, so the lesson was learned. I remember that I did not cry because of the slap and bore it stoically, my classmates thinking I was naughty but very brave!

Some of the most interesting lessons involved using our hands and being creative. Every now and again the school caretaker Mr Murgatroyd, a formidable figure wearing a grey overall, would appear in the classroom just before dinner bringing with him a big galvanised steel bin with a tight fitting lid, inside which was a large piece of very cold modelling clay. We looked forward to Mr Murgatroyd's visit to the classroom, and knew that when we came back that afternoon we could muck about to our hearts' content making 'things'. I always tried to make a railway engine, I'd finished with buses by this time, having been on the train on the annual Sunday school outing to Hunstanton, and was now a convert to the railway and all its works. And I discovered that I wasn't sick on a train!

This visit to Hunstanton was a regular and much looked forward to yearly event. We went by a specially chartered train along with other Sunday schools in the area. The day started at about 7.00am; we all walked down to the chapel where we were labelled with a brown cardboard label, and if you objected to being thus labelled you either got a clip round the ear or it was threatened that you would be sent home to bed, told to 'stop moaning and enjoy yourself'. The next thing was a prayer from the minister asking for journeying mercies, whatever they were, another problem to think about. We then traipsed down to the station a mile away behind a flag and waited with great excitement to see a wisp of steam up the cutting as the first sign that the train was coming.

We arrived after the most exiting journey of some two hours later at Hunstanton station, detrained, and as a group formed a crocodile and marched down to the beach behind the minister who was carrying the large union flag. We found ourselves a spot on the beach, around the flag of course, and proceeded to unpack the sardine sandwiches and bottles of Tizer provided for us by Mum, and not until we had eaten our fill were we allowed to go for a paddle, being told 'and don't fall in!' this was sometimes not so easy as the tide at Hunstanton went out a long way, leaving huge mud flats, much to our disappointment!

Tea was provided by the minister, and about 4.00pm we all paraded before him, tidied ourselves up and marched into the town behind the flag to a café where we were expected, and served sandwiches and cup cakes by young waitresses dressed in black with white aprons and frilly lace caps.

We all sat down very sedately, and the minister started the meal with grace. The trouble was he used a verse of a hymn for this purpose, and we were told off if we didn't sing even though we didn't know the tune or the words!

After this gourmet repast, we tidied up, marched back to the station to catch the train, arriving back at Letchworth about 7.00pm. Back at the chapel we took off our labels; these were collected to be used again next year! And with a valedictory prayer of thanks for our journeying mercies, which we had apparently received, went home tired but happy; we'd seen the sea again! And so straight to bed.

As a family we were not well off, of course, nobody was in those days. One morning sitting on the floor in morning assembly in which we expressed our gratitude to God for another day to work and play in, I started to cry with the pain in my heel. I had outgrown my shoes; Father had tried to stretch them before, after hammering studs in to make them last longer, but they had rubbed the skin off my delicate extremities causing a blister which had burst. A teacher took me to the staff room where she anointed the raw area with neat iodine solution, not exactly a comfortable procedure; she put some dressing on and gave me a note to take home to Mum.

The outcome of this event was a visit to the Coop and the purchase of a pair of new shoes, but these had square toes. So far as I was concerned, comfortable they may have been, shoes did not in my experience have square toes and that was that, and I was not going to wear them, so there! This resulted in another slap; life was getting hard!

Then my Mackintosh was too small, I was a growing lad, another visit to the Coop. Don't let us forget, this earned divvy points I was told, whatever they were, but the new mack was voluminous, being a cheap one that was made of some sort of oiled silk, and I hated it! Macks were not made of that stuff, and it was a greenish colour. Macks to me were blue and made of cloth. Another admonishment was forthcoming as a result of my rebellion, but the first time I had to wear it on a rainy cold morning, as I went out of the back door I took it off and left it on the step, and walked the three hundred yards to school in only my jumper and arrived soaked to the skin, resulting in another serious telling off, and a streaming cold!

The first year of my academic career went reasonably well; we were after all only learning to live together with a smattering of rote learning thrown in, as was the technique in those days, and each day finished with a story. That was great and we always looked forward to it, particularly the one about the tiger that chased its own tail and got faster and faster until it melted into a dish of butter. Why I should remember that one I don't know, it must have been the expertise of the narrator or something!

Sunday was the day we were supposed to behave differently. Sunday school in the afternoon was taught by various members of the chapel, who felt it was their duty to teach the kids right from wrong. It was again, for us youngsters, a time of stories, not always so expertly told as at day school, but bible stories which would appeal to young minds interspersed with chorus singing which tried to give a smattering of theology in them. I enjoyed the singing even if I didn't understand the words or the message they were designed to convey! Some of the tunes were very catchy and remain with me today. One I particularly liked was 'Whither pilgrim are you going, going each with staff in hand, we are going on a journey, going to a better land'. But I did like the idea of the journey! I didn't know it, but I was just starting mine. I wasn't sure about this better land; the present one as a much loved child seemed to me to be alright anyway. This was a throwback to the old Victorian scene of child labour and deprivation I learned later, but it took me many years to unravel the theology behind it all. It was all too much for a child's brain, a bit dodgy for an adult in this day and age! And we still have not understood that heaven on Earth – this better land – could be achieved if we all behaved ourselves.

Sunday school lessons must have been effective to some extent, the concept of sin was always being taught. Looking back on this, having never been given a definition of sin (on reflection in my eightieth year), I eventually came to the sad conclusion that sin was anything the teachers, church authorities or our parents didn't approve of! And retribution was the natural consequence of this wrongdoing, but we never did get hold of the idea that any wrongdoing was forgiven if we were repentant and said sorry, and tried to make amends. This resulted one day at day school, coming home after classes one evening, I discovered to my absolute horror that I had by accident brought home a school pencil, I convinced myself that was stealing! I really was appalled at my behavior, but was unable to understand that I could right the wrong by taking it back the following morning, so I went to the bottom of the garden, dug a hole and buried the evidence of my crime before it was discovered by the authorities! It is probably still there to this day but I didn't dare tell my parents of my fall from grace!

It was there at Sunday school that I learnt the words. I didn't understand them at the time, but the words were to stay with me all my life buried deep in my memory. It was later in my life that as I brought them to mind with the experiences of life, I found out what they really meant, the ideas of loving your neighbour, caring for the weaker in society, compassion for the sick, self-control, responsibility. No, not just words, but the very essence of life as it should be led in a civilised society. These words were the building blocks, which have enabled me to build a worthwhile life and to spend it caring for others.

There were other horrors and pitfalls on the bill for the young attempting to fit in with this world of academia at school.

School toilets were not exactly up to the super loo standard of today, but adequate. My great problem at this age was not undoing the buttons of my braces so that I could drop my trousers to perform, it was the doing up afterwards when I was ready that caused the difficulty. I could not do up the back buttons, and would spend ages in the toilet until the worried teacher came to investigate my prolonged absence from class. Why in heaven's name I didn't have the wit just to slip the braces over my shoulders I will never know; it took me some time to realise that this was the logical way to do it. As it was, if I did manage to do up the buttons, I would then get the braces twisted and on return to the class spend ages fidgeting around in sheer discomfort until I was put out of my misery by my exasperated teacher, and told off in the presence of the whole class, and just stood there to have my clothing sorted out!

Ahead were other hazards and terrors for the uninitiated. We were learning in a very simple way a subject called nature study. There was a teacher who would bring into her lessons such things as dead mice and other examples of wild life, and one day she had been to the local pond near her house and had brought some denizens of the deep for us to look at. She had found the larvae of the common dragonfly which we were to marvel over. I didn't like the appearance of these, to me, bizarre creatures, and found them for some reason quite threatening, and after class I developed an earache of some intensity and was convinced that one of these larvae had jumped out of its jar and got into my ear and was eating away into my brain to its heart's content. I ran home to Mother crying until she discovered the reason for my fears, and like a good mother she was able to put these fears to rest with the usual treatment in those days, love and a few drops of hot olive oil in the ear canal, which did the trick!

Other major events occurred, particularly before the Christmas holiday when the school decided to give a concert for the parents. This consisted of a sort of dissertation on the British weather, and the bit I was to be in was concerned with the winds of Autumn. This was to demonstrate the powerful effects of the wind blowing on the trees. The 'trees' would sing a sort of protest song about how it could blow all the leaves around, but I was not chosen to be a tree to wear a costume like a tree trunk with leaves coming out of the head. Much to my utter disgust, I had to be a member of the choir that sang 'Have you seen the wind' etc.; I remember the tune to this day! But I wanted to be a tree; my best friend Alex was a tree, so why wasn't I? Was that fair? But then, I was made to wear a white shirt and white trouser and white sandals so it wasn't too bad after all, but not as good as being a tree!

By now there were noises abroad of international friction. Father came home and talked about the crisis and fighting a war. I couldn't get my head round that one, but both parents were obviously worried about this thing called a crisis. I can understand now how devastating it must have been for them to anticipate another war, it was after all only twenty or so years since they had to live through the previous one, but from now on it seemed to me that all the grownups could talk about was this strange thing called a crisis, and look worried when it was discussed or read about in the newspapers.

However, it did seem to blow over, but a strange new intake of children began to arrive at the school with funny names, who could not speak English very well. We were told by our teacher to be very kind to these kids because some of them had lost their parents in a country called Germany, but like all kids we fell out with them as much as we fell out with each other! Also they were called Jews, we'd heard about them from the bible, but they didn't look anything like those Jews such as Goliath or King David or Saul whose pictures we'd seen in the illustrated bible that we had at home!

Most of these foreign kids were living in the local orphanage called Briar Patch, and would walk home in a gang after school. They became a favourite target for the other estate children, until we learned to our cost that one of these newcomers, a bit bigger than the rest, called Jacob, could throw stones more accurately than us, the home grown product. So thereafter they were left alone!

In the summer of the following year, not long after our annual holiday to Clacton, the 'crisis' returned. We were rudely awakened one morning with the wailing of the air raid siren, the first time I'd heard it. I thought at first it was a wild animal which had escaped and was roaming the streets. I looked out the window to see the fire brigade tender in position in the event of a bomb dropping, but it was a false alarm, and so the country went to war, and our lives were never the same again. Then another lot of children descended on us called evacuees, mainly from London, they brought even funnier ways with them than Jacob's lot! They really were streetwise, these kids, and got up to all kinds of mischief!

Now all kinds of strange things began to happen; our playing field next to the school was suddenly turned into a huge building site, but the builders were building it under the ground. We were told it was all about air raid precautions; things like that were only briefly explained to us. We were told that aeroplanes would drop bombs which would blow us all up. We found that a bit difficult; most of us hadn't ever seen an aeroplane. Yes, we'd seen pictures of them, but they didn't look dangerous. Later we were to learn how dangerous they were; when the air raid sirens sounded we were forced to sit in these shelters for hours at a time, and the bombers came over and we heard the rumble of their engines and the crump of exploding bombs somewhere distant. To pass the time we sat and sang such classics as 'Three Green Bottles' and 'One Man Went to Mow' and so on to take our minds off the cold and damp of these underground tunnels, fun at first, but they gradually lost their allure when no bombs dropped near us; and of course, the holiday in Clacton was cancelled. That really hurt!

Slowly the seriousness of the situation became clearer to us as we heard the news on the BBC and were shown pictures in the paper of what war was about, and our interest was aroused, and in my case trains gave way to Spitfires in my life, and I wanted to fly one!

We were issued with gas masks and had to take them with us everywhere we went, because 'you know what these Germans are like, they used gas in the last war and wouldn't hesitate to use it on us now,' we were told. So we had to learn to put them on quickly; we were told that in the event of a gas attack the ARP warden would come round the street shouting 'Gas! Gas!', swinging a rattle, and we were to drop whatever we were doing and comply immediately. There was no time to waste. We had to practice putting on the gas masks of course, but certain members of the family were slower than others and my younger brother, about three years old at this time, objected strongly to having his face buried in this unsightly rubber monstrosity and yelled his head off. It required the full energy of both parents to force it over his head. My query was, 'how can we eat our dinner wearing one of those?' The question was treated with the contempt it deserved, and I was told to shut up or else! However, as we never needed to wear them as the risk of invasion receded, they became a bit more rubbish with which to clutter the house.

School continued, the holidays in the summer and at Christmas were shortened, the government thought it best to have children in recognisable places and as we could no longer travel anywhere like the seaside, one assumes they didn't think it a good idea to have hoards of children roaming the streets.

Father, at this time being too old to be called up into the army, was informed that he would be directed to a job concerned with war work and went to work in a scientific instrument factory in the town. The wages were better than he had received whilst working in the shop repairing watches, but for all the extra income, goods were disappearing off the shelves and there was less to buy as the whole economy geared up to win the war.

As children we didn't really understand what was going on, and continued to muck about and get whatever fun we could out of life, but certain events cast long shadows over our lives making everybody sad and worried, such as the evacuation from Dunkirk, and later the surrender of Singapore – my parents had a friend whose son was there at the time. The sinking of the battleships off Malaya as Japan joined the war also caused much grief.

My elder brother at this time informed me that in the future anybody who owned any toys made in Japan would be bombed, resulting in me scavenging around in my toy box looking frantically for a small tinplate racing car which I knew I had somewhere and was made in Japan. I consigned this to the dustbin with alacrity when I found it!

These were the nights of the blackout. All windows were covered with black curtains to avoid any chink of light being shown. A lit cigarette could be seen from ten thousand feet, we were told, and the blackout was rigorously enforced; anyone showing a light at night could be a spy. The windows were also crisscrossed with brown paper strips to lessen the effect of blast injuries from bombing, which would result in shards of glass flying around. Brick blast walls were built to shield certain downstairs rooms from blast injury; our kitchen was deemed the most vulnerable room, so it was always dark. But you had no choice; any deviation from regulations and you were looked on as uncooperative and suspect.

All in all we were slowly being confined within a huge set of regulations against which there was no appeal. We knew when things were getting really bad, an announcement would be made on the BBC that the king would be addressing the nation that evening; he would give a brief resume of the state of the nation and the war, and then announce that the following week there would be a day of prayer and all citizens were encouraged to find a local church and join in; and then the prime minister, a Mr Winston Churchill, would address the nation, pulling no punches, and encourage us all to work for eventual victory which would be ours because our cause was just! His very voice, even to we children, was uplifting, and at the end of his speech my dad used to cheer.

Father in the meantime had become a fire watcher, an official group of men who spent part of the night in shifts preparing for fire bomb raids – this was the time of the blitz in London. We were only about thirty miles from London and we would see the sky lit up night after night with the flames as London burned, and we could hear the constant rumble of bombs falling throughout the night. Sometimes the bombers would overshoot the city and unload their bombs into our surrounding countryside, we as a family then spent the night under the living room table huddled together wondering what was going to happen next. My main complaint about this was that my elder brother had smelly feet which I objected to, and I was quite voluble with my complaint until told to shut up. Once I was told that to die moaning about his feet would never get me to heaven!

Father then joined the Home Guard. We were very proud of him in his uniform, and when he brought home his Sten gun, well that was awesome. He and his colleagues would charge around on exercises in the town looking war-like; I don't know if they would have frightened the enemy, but they had a good time, all together in the war effort. He used to come home with stories of the exercises they had, and we listened enthralled to these stories of rifle shooting, and the use of thunderflashes which made a huge bang. Quite illegally he brought one home with him one Sunday morning after exercise, it had refused to go off when thrown at 'the enemy' and he set it off in the back garden with a slow burning fuse, which resulted in a visit from the police querying what had caused the explosion. Some jealous neighbour reported it I assume!

By this time food was getting in short supply and the ingenuity of my mother in feeding us was taxed to the limit, we grew a few vegetables in the garden, but with the war work and other jobs my father had little time for gardening. I had a go and promptly nearly severed the tip of my thumb by sharpening a hoe because I thought it would be a better tool and remove more weeds, so I took a file out of father's tool kit and got to work to end up with a massive haemorrhage from my nearly severed index finger, resulting in a trip to the doctor, which of course cost more money, and I got moaned at for my pains.

Meat was rationed by the amount it cost, a shilling's worth would buy so much liver, so much beef, so much lamb. There was rarely pork unless you knew someone who was in a pig club, as it was known, and raised a pig feeding it on kitchen scraps until it was ready for slaughter, and then all members of the club got a bit and the government got half! By the time we got to Wednesday, most of the meat of any type had been used up and we were left with a small piece of scragg end of mutton, which was boiled with onions. I couldn't stand it and would heave when it was put in front of me for dinner with the admonition, 'there's nothing else, eat it or go without', and if I complained too much, I would get a clip round the ear and sent to bed as soon as I came in from school. I was also advised to think of all the little children in France who had even less under the occupation. Good for them, I recall thinking; at least they don't get boiled mutton!

Everything now was directed to the war effort. We had frequent 'war weapons weeks' where a Spitfire or a crashed Messerschmitt, and even once a mini submarine, made by a local factory which before the war made dustcarts, was on display in the town, with the intention of attracting the public to invest in war bonds or national savings certificates to further the war effort. We greatly loved these very exciting exhibitions, where crowds of curious onlookers attended and we were allowed to sit in the aircraft or pretend to operate their guns, usually demonstrated to us by servicemen in uniform. Crashed German aircraft were often on show and mobile cinemas showed such propaganda films as *Target for Tonight*, which showed some of the huge raids which the Allied forces were now flying over enemy territory.

A great source of collectables formed a thriving market for we kids in unrecognisable bits and pieces of what we were assured were genuine aircraft parts, and changed hands by 'swaps' frequently.

There was a dog fight over the town one night. A night fighter caught a German intruder bomber and shot it down, the aircraft crashed some ten miles away, but the town and surrounding fields were littered with shell cases, which we, against all regulations and warnings, collected and hid away from our parents.

One member of the most anti-social family in the street found a live cannon shell. They were not of the brightest intellects, that family; the father took it to work the next day, and in the foundry of the factory where he worked attempted to explode it, and in the process lost two fingers of his right hand. This event was widely published as a warning to all to leave things alone if we found anything suspicious.

Our own minor contribution to the war was to trawl around the streets with an old pram and collect what were euphemistically called 'comforts for the troops at the front'. These comforts were anything from old bits of clothing – preferably woollen knitwear, which could be unravelled and reformed as balacalava helmets for the Russians – to old aluminium pots and pans to make aeroplanes, and of course books. I think that this was where I developed my love of books even at this young age. We were quite naughty and took out anything that looked interesting and readable for ourselves, before handing the rest of the goodies over to the collecting centre which was in the old gospel hall next to the library. I found some wonderful books such as Jules Verne's *The English At the North Pole*, *Twenty Thousand Leagues under The Sea* and a Mark Twain gem called *A Tramp Abroad*, which I still have in my possession today. These opened a whole new world for me, having been brought up on Sunday school prize books which by no stretch of the imagination exercised one's mind at all in any direction, being mainly about well-behaved and well-intentioned children from upper-class families living in superior houses with a cook and gardener, who looked after the kitchen and garden, did their bit for the poor and needy, and helped old ladies cross the road! But my time in school was reasonably productive and I could by now read and write fairly well and began to take an interest in books, having collected so many round the streets.

My older brother by this time was becoming quite an accomplished pianist, and it was suggested that I should now start piano lessons with the same teacher. But it was now getting towards the time when I had to think about the future. My brother had left the junior school, and was attending the secondary school at the other end of the town and had to cycle there each day, but my father was thinking of better things for me, and government plans were afoot to offer assisted places for grammar school education for those who passed the entrance exam. This was not going to happen in the near future, but was on the cards, and the government was thinking ahead to post-war reconstruction as news from the front line eased. So I started music lessons. These were arranged for a Saturday afternoon and involved a walk to the other side of the town to be taught by the same teacher my brother studied under. The trouble with this plan was that everything I did in future would be compared to my brother's prowess, but I had a go and I'm afraid I could not find the enthusiasm that he had, and so did not progress according to my parents' plan, much to their disappointment. However, sad to relate, I think it was the aversion I had to the teacher. She had a funny smell about her! She did not appeal to me at all and I would often find a subject not associated with music to talk about, so I had little time to play the work I had been given to practice the week before, and she, poor woman, fell for it each time!

Each Saturday afternoon we would walk up this long, long road to the teacher's house. Her house was on the right side of the road at the end of a block. But my brother for some reason always insisted that when we got to within a hundred yards of the house, we crossed the road to the opposite side. On that side, at the point where the houses finished, the cottage hospital gardens began. In the garden right next to the footpath was a small vent for the sewage system for the road. It had a grill in the front, and my brother told me that in there all the bad tonsils that were removed from the patients at the hospital were placed after they'd been removed, and if we breathed in as we went past it we would get a dreadful disease and die, so we had to hold our breath and run past as fast as we could or we'd be in trouble. I fell for this and felt I had to comply with his instructions – after all he was very clever and older than I – so ended up at the teacher's house blue in the face and completely out of breath. I was about eight at the time, so why I believed this nonsense I really don't know, but it did not increase my enthusiasm for music lessons!

By that time I was almost in the top class at school. The new education act that had been rumoured was passed by Parliament, but as I was about to be coached for the grammar school, I fell ill with a serious abdominal complaint which scuppered all thoughts of the future for the time being, and indeed postponed my father's plans for me by some eighteen months.

One evening on return from school, my mother found me sitting hunched up in a chair – quite unusual for me, I was a very active child and would normally be out messing about and having a good time.

I was complaining of vague abdominal pain and feeling unwell. This rapidly developed into severe pain with vomiting and the doctor was sent for. The doctor was an immigrant who had escaped Nazi persecution, and was reputed to be a very clever man, and being a Jew, my parents thinking was that they were doing God's work in patronising the needy and oppressed, changed over to his panel of patients as it was known in those days.

However he obviously didn't know how to deal with my problem and allowed it to develop to the point where I was desperately ill. Another doctor from the same practice was called and I was immediately whisked off to hospital where I was operated on for a perforated appendix with subsequent peritonitis the same evening; and so began for me three months of misery with my life hanging on a thread. Most of the time I was unaware of what was happening, apart from two more drainage operations to drain the pus from pelvic abscesses. In the end the corner was turned by a transfusion of my father's blood, which set me on the road to recovery. These days with antibiotics, it would have got no further than a bellyache, but there was nothing that could be done before these wonderful drugs were available. Another child in the same road died with the same problem some weeks later, and she had been operated on promptly. In those days you often went to hospital to die.

Then started a long period of convalescence, away from school for over a year and being treated with kid gloves!

However, I'd missed a year's schooling and had to be told that my chances of the grammar school were now put back, and I would have to stay at my junior school for another year, this was a bit devastating because all my friends had moved on and I was with a new set of children. I did eventually enter for the scholarship exam to go to grammar school and promptly failed, and had to wait another year until I could take the new exam for an assisted place, which was now available because of the passing of the 1944 Education Act!

So I was now all set to go to this prestigious new school. Things were changing internationally; the second front had occurred and the Allies were winning, but the enemy still had not finished with us and the time of the flying bombs arrived, and once again we spent time under the living room table, listening to the awful *throb throb* of these infernal machines and waiting for the engine to stop, then the agonising silence, wondering if it would hit us as we waited for the explosion. Fortunately none fell in our town, but did in the surrounding fields, and devastated a village some four miles distant.

4

THE NEW WORLD OF THE GRAMMAR SCHOOL

So the very exciting time came for the purchase of the new school uniform, and for the first time I would be wearing long trousers. This really was a rite of passage in those days, showing that you were growing up and joining the adult world! I was only allowed one set of clothes; they were rationed and cost not only money but clothing coupons. The number you were allowed depended upon your circumstances. There was of course an enhanced allowance for special things such as going to a new school, but I also had to have P.E. kit and should have had football boots, but that proved too expensive in money and clothing coupons for us at that time. I remember wearing the uniform for the first time; I was so proud and indeed so were my parents; I had to wear it to chapel the Sunday before I started at my new school and it was much admired by all.

But of course, with a very queasy feeling in my stomach, Monday morning came round all too soon and I had to start what I felt was a completely new life.

The school was about three times larger than my old junior school, and peopled by such exalted figures as prefects, and school masters in academic gowns and hoods, all so strange to me in my innocence.

There was a lot of noise and people rushing around and telling us what to do, and to do it quietly and immediately. We started in the hall with an assembly – the hall was to be called big school from now on – sang a hymn, had a couple of prayers by the headmaster, an imposing figure at a desk on the rostrum with the rest of the staff on parade, then we were welcomed along with all the others to the new term and then names were called out, along with such mysteries as Smith major and Smith minor. We had never heard this kind of appellation before! Then we were allocated to our class and classroom. I was allocated to 1b, not quite as good as 1a, but we felt we were better than those allocated to 1c, where all the duffers went, so we were told!

The teachers were of a different calibre to those we had known in our junior school, as indeed were the kids themselves. Most in those days were from middle-class families, and it was the 1944 Education Act which gave easier access to the grammar school system to kids like me from the council estates. However my father still had to pay something to the authorities for my education; a small fee, but it was a sacrifice even though with war work he was being paid more than when he worked in a shop.

The subjects taught were different; we now had algebra, trigonometry, geometry, as well as the usual geography, and history, and if this was not enough to tax our bemused minds, French and Latin, which really caused us problems, mainly I think because the teacher was a small, unsmiling and demanding man and any misconduct resulted in the culprit having to spend the rest of the lesson standing in the waste paper basket in the corner facing the wall – and if that wasn't punishment enough, half an hour's detention after school where we had to do mathematics, guaranteed to put you off a subject for life! But we soon shook down and found our level; we were expected to be able to answer questions put to us and not just cringe down behind the boy in front, to give reasoned replies to questions, and to think before we spoke. No longer were we to be spoon-fed, but we had to take some responsibility for our actions.

I did not enjoy the experience initially, but soldiered on hoping for it all to get easier. With the resilience of youth I coped, even though I was still getting problems with my medical problem which still caused me pain at times, and required a note to the headmaster for me to be excused whatever strenuous activity was planned for us.

The school played rugby football and the doctors had suggested that this activity was best avoided for me, but of course among children anybody who was different was looked on with suspicion and taunted about it if possible.

There were one or two subjects which helped to restore my self esteem, which was taking a battering from the clever and upper-class kids I had to live with. One such subject was music. The teacher of this subject always had a kind word for me for some reason. The first session where all the class were gathered in the music room was a getting to know you session. Miss Lyons, the teacher – she got married later to the senior maths master and became Mrs Bentley – asked if any of us had had music lessons. One young man, whose father was in the Salvation Army band, straight away announced proudly that he was learning the piano. This opened the conversation a bit and one or two others said that they had in the past. Miss Lyons then opened a hymn book on the piano and asked anyone who could play to demonstrate their prowess. The young S.A. boy immediately had a go and did very badly I thought. I had not admitted to the ability to play then as I wanted to see what the others could do. The tune was a well-known one, the old German anthem by Hadyn. This was four part harmony, and one thing I had learned to do was to play hymn tunes, although I had given up lessons. So when the teacher asked if there was anyone else who wanted to play, I volunteered to have a go, much to the amusement of the class in which I was not a popular member. I sat down and played it note perfect with aplomb! Miss Lyons was impressed and told me that I had a very good touch for my age, and so developed a friendship that lasted whilst I was at the school, and put a few of my fellow pupils' noses out of joint!

Miss Lyons did her best with this rather intellectual wilderness of young adolescents; a few of us appreciated what she was trying to do, but it must have been an uphill struggle in those days before music was as common as it later became with easy access to concerts, on radio and T.V.

In fact I continued to study music theory with her for the rest of my time at school. We even went to recitals by famous pianists who performed locally. I eventually took the subject in my school certificate exams when I finished my time there and got a good grade. The other subject I excelled at was what was known as drawing, or art. I drew a magnificent picture of a Spitfire which was much admired by my colleagues, but did not progress much further than that! The teacher didn't like me and I couldn't stand her, the feeling was mutual I'm afraid!

By this time the music scene in the town was getting going, at the local big nonconformist church know as the Free Church, the choirmaster decided that he would have an augmented choir from various organisations and churches in the town, to perform Handel's Messiah each year at Easter.

He invited various well-known national artists to perform, and within a few years the performance became the annual music event of the year in the town, and when a very famous organist, Dr Eric Thiman, was invited to accompany the annual performance, it really took off.

My elder brother by this time was doing very well musically and turned his sights on the organ. He began to take organ lessons from the choirmaster, and after a couple of years asked if he could sit with this famous organist and turn the pages for him as he played Messiah. This was a moment of great pride to us. Mother was in the choir by now, and eventually some years later, my brother took lessons from the great man and played in his stead. He progressed from this, and eventually after a lot of hard work and study at university, became a Fellow of the Royal College of Organists and joined the greats.

One other aspect of our lives concerned with music was my elder brother's formation of an all-girls choir. This proved to be very popular, and although he confined the numbers to twelve members, there were always those who wanted to join. The criteria was their ability to sing, of course, but he did the selection, and he did end up with a very good looking lot of young ladies. I suspect that their looks played some part in the selection process! I was involved in a minor way when I sat next to him at the piano and turned the pages of the music. We had one or two rather prestigious occasions when the choir sang at some of the big houses in the area, and a number of dinners where we used to entertain after the meal. Both my brother and I had to be dressed properly for these occasions and we both wore black coats and striped trousers which looked, and made me feel, very superior! Once we even got our picture taken and put in the local paper! We also, and this was the best of the lot, went carol singing at Christmas, and were sometimes invited in for a refresher before we moved on. All in all, a good time was had by all with many happy memories.

It was, however, still wartime with all its restrictions, and we were still encouraged to do our bit for the war effort. The schools were asked to provide labour to go potato picking, as it was known, or as we called it 'spud bashing'.

We were picked up at school by a bus and taken to a local farm where we were expected to pick up the potatoes after they had been lifted by the machine. Each of we kids was given a pitch, and as the tractor came round lifting all the potatoes, we collected them and put them in trugs which were then collected by another tractor and trailer. We had to wear our scruffiest clothes for this, every now and again a mobile canteen would arrive driven by WVS volunteers who dispensed hot drinking chocolate, which was free. We enjoyed that, and looked forward to the visit of the van as a break in the monotony from picking up spuds for some six hours. It was quite back-breaking work and we were not allowed to talk to our neighbours as we worked, and for this labour were paid the princely sum of one shilling a session, quite a good wage to a teenager in those days. It certainly made a break from school and lessons, but most of us caught colds because we would take our coats off as the other farm workers did, and we didn't want to be different.

We now moved to another bigger house on the estate, and I had a bedroom of my own, which was rather nice. I used to lay in bed at night, my room being directly over the 'front room' where my brother used to practice the piano for hours at a time. I still remember one piece, burned into my memory, 'The Golliwog's Cake Walk'. He went on and on until he got it right, sometimes up to midnight, when my parents had had enough and stopped him, but his success later in life was due to his constant practice.

One other lesson I enjoyed was art. We had various teachers; mostly gentle people, but one woman was a bit of a harridan and for some reason took a dislike to me. One of the most serious punishments that were handed out to any of us considered to be an 'extremely disruptive element' was a special detention which involved firstly your name being put in a special black book, kept I believe in the headmaster's study. This was nasty as it resulted in a one hour detention with something like a series of Latin verbs to deal with. I ended up in this for no other reason than this teacher thought I had said something rude to her, when in fact it was my neighbour who had been the culprit. The teacher would not listen to what I said, and my colleague would not own up. I was therefore told to report after school to the appropriate room to do my sentence the following day. We had been told that twelve entries in this book would result in our expulsion from the school, and to not attend was the gravest crime in the book.

But I didn't attend, feeling a great sense of injustice, and the next morning at assembly, my name was called out to see the head at two o'clock. I was aware of the seriousness of this crime and expected a severe punishment, and spent the morning in absolute terror. However, when I got home for dinner at the end of the morning, relief was at hand, outside the house was the big cream coloured fever ambulance which was carting my younger brother off to the isolation hospital with diphtheria. I was dragged indoors, a throat swab was taken and we were all, including our parents, confined to a week's quarantine, and the house was fumigated with some form of gas. I can recall the comment of the workman who did this; he'd done one the previous week and there were still spiders alive in the house when he'd finished, he claimed, so thought it was a waste of time!

So on return to school a week later, nothing more was said about the black book detention, thanks to my brother's disease. It was a nasty disease and the poor chap spent three months in the fever hospital, and of the thirteen children in the street who were incarcerated with him, three died from the complications of the disease, but I'd got away without a severe reprimand or worse because of my brother's misfortune. I must remember to thank him some time!

We were slowly winning this war and life became easier. The blackout was lifted slightly and we began to live in hope that a good future awaited the country. But all attitudes did not change; there was a feeling around that we deserved to win because we were not so wicked as the Germans, who were spawns of Satan to say the least about them!

We had studied history at a different level and could see, and were expected to see, parallels between events in history and our own present day situation. The concept that might be right was considered to be the mainstream view of life, but not necessarily true.

I was still attending Sunday school, although I was told I would be going to join a youth organisation called the Covenanters when I was fourteen, which in reality only turned out to be an extension of the ideas given us at the Sunday school, the difference being that the members were older, and the local leader of this group was a pacifist. I recall showing him a picture of the Spitfire I had drawn, to be told in no uncertain terms that this was an evil machine designed to kill people and had no place in my thoughts. There was brooked no argument about this, but by now there was a growing dichotomy in my beliefs which worried me. It had been rammed into us that the Kingdom of Heaven consisted only of those good people who believed what we did! During a question and answer session with the leaders of the various youth groups I posed the question that I had been taught at school that it had taken many million years for the world to develop to where we were today, and the bible said it was formed in six days – what was I to believe? I was very quickly shot down in flames and was told that I should pray for enlightenment and indeed they would pray for me in my apostasy!

I was also told that I should make a stand for what I believed, and be baptised, and join the church and have all my thoughts and direction in life guided by prayer and reading of good books. At that time I wasn't sure just what I did believe!

One day when the minister visited us, a book belonging to my elder brother was lying on a chair. It was a novel about the American Civil War. The minister picked it up and told him to get rid of it as it was unsuitable reading for the young. My brother was furious, and when he proceeded to argue was told by Mother to behave himself and never ever talk to the minister like that again, in her eyes the minister was equated with the Almighty if not the Almighty himself! Not long after this episode my poor brother was again hauled over the coals. Some interfering busybody saw that he had one day parked his bike outside the local cinema. The fact that he couldn't find room for it in the cycle rack outside the public library was dismissed, the verdict was guilty, he must have been to the cinema! Oh these people!

This of course began to grate, this everlasting lambasting of anything that the chapel didn't either understand or agree with. Never any concession to the thought that you might have a point of view, and let's have a look at it. But fundamentalism was ingrained in these people, and some of the most intelligent people would put accepted knowledge aside, and subscribe to their agreed text as they knew it was true! So they claimed! However, they were very good people at heart and had your best interests as their main concern. Misguided they may have been, either unwilling or unable to see that their ideas did not always equate with even common sense, but to me I failed to see if it mattered whether the world did or did not take millions of years to create. Also, what did it matter if Christmas day fell on a Sunday, and then to cap it all, you were denied your presents until Monday? That seemed to me to make a mockery of the whole spirit of the festival! When I did have the temerity to comment upon these thoughts I was usually put down with the kind but withering remark that 'We'll pray for you, for your enlightenment and awareness of the truth'. This of course, I soon realised, was not for my benefit, but so that I would see things their way and accept the concepts of the medieval world that their minds seemed to inhabit and in which they were comfortable, and so not upset them.

I can recall some years later a boyhood friend of mine with whom I had kept in contact over the years, when he learned that I, now a fifty-year-old man, was studying acupuncture, refused thereafter to have anything to do with me, as sticking needles in people was the devil's work! Why I did not lose my faith in God after all this, I can only put down to the goodness of God, who gave me a brain to use, and eyes to see, and ears to hear!

They all seemed unable to comprehend that it wasn't the protocol you followed that mattered, but what you were; that is, how you behaved to your fellow man, no matter what his condition or beliefs, and to treat others as you would wish to be treated yourself, the golden rule as expressed by Christ himself.

It also seemed to me as I got older, that to these people, it wasn't only what you did that mattered, but in particular what you did not do that would earn you brownie points, and the things that you did not do were numerous, and these were chiefly things in which you would get maximum enjoyment, such as going to football matches and the cinema or theatre. In fact I was fifteen years old before I went to a cinema, and to my shame had to tell lies to achieve this, but to sit in the auditorium and be entertained by a tale of derring do did not surely by any stretch of the imagination forbid me entrance one day in the distant future to this Kingdom of Heaven! I can recall at this time a rather po-faced uncle of mine observing that what an appalling thing it would be if on the return of Christ to claim his kingdom on earth, I was found at a football match. His response to my glib reply that if he did, he'd probably join in and have a kick around with us was not only blasphemy, but not the way to think, and I was destined for hell if that was my attitude! And of course he would pray for me! This was of course a real throwback to the puritan movement of the seventeenth century.

Your whole attitude was to be humble, and to be proud of it! Certainly not to enjoy the life you had been given. But Sunday school had its moments, some embarrassing and literally painful to a young lad. There were two events held regularly each year; not in the chapel, because it was too small, but in other locations in the town. These were the Sunday school anniversary celebrations and the prize giving, into both of which you were usually dragooned to perform in some way before an audience, to your utter terror.

The anniversary was in reality no more than another service to which all the parents of the scholars, many being non-churchgoers, who only sent the kids to Sunday school to get them out of the way on a Sunday afternoon, were invited, and the preacher billed as 'a special speaker' which I assume was designed to encourage attendance at the event. This august personage could be anyone of note in the chapel movement, but he was also someone of local importance and socially superior to most of us. Most of the children, because of the location of the chapel, were of working-class parents, but the leading lights of the organisation were mainly white-collar workers. None of them, if I can recall, were trained theologians or even teachers, so their message was often the same, and to we children, boring in the extreme, and not understood anyway. I think the service was really to show off what an erudite lot they were, the speakers always from the better off part of society who came to the service in a motor car, a real badge of distinction in those far off days! I recall in the later days of the war, the 'special speaker' was a Lt. Colonel no less, who was fawned upon as though he was a relative of the king himself!

But for us kids, the terror was that we would be chosen to perform something such as a recitation or the reading of a psalm to the audience, and we had no option but to do it; it was expected of you, if you did not comply you paid the price when you got home!

For my sins, one anniversary I had to stand on the stage of the hall and accompany a song with tubular bells, but with some of my day school friends in the audience, who were there with their parents and did not attend Sunday school, I was totally mortified and was not allowed to forget it.

The prize giving was held in a big hall above the main Coop shop in the town. Much the same type of event, and one time when much younger, I was made to sing a duet to the audience with a friend of mine, Johnny Fitch, a small cherubic-faced boy with a cheeky grin. We started to sing this rubbish of three verses as a duet, but after the first line my companion decided not to continue and I had to struggle along on my own, and he just stood there grinning. Afterwards I asked him why he'd left me in the lurch, and he replied he didn't like the song anyway, and that was that!

However, after all the performances and the sermon from the 'special speaker' we got to the prizes, usually one for attendance and another for good behaviour or for something you had done which was worth a few brownie points. Everybody got a prize however; nobody was allowed to go without! The books were hardly out of the top drawer of the literary canon, but they were free even if we did not read them, but my parents thought they were 'lovely books' and we were very honoured to have them presented to us by the minister himself!

Then one day, just after my fourteenth birthday, the war did end. We knew from the news that things were going to happen, and one glorious day there was a lot of shouting on the streets. 'It's all over!' We all tumbled out of the house to celebrate.

The King and Mr Churchill broadcast to the nation on the BBC, and great was the rejoicing with street parties, parades and other ceremonies to celebrate the victory. The sense of relief was palpable, but it was soon tinged with pity by those who thought seriously of what had happened, so many millions uprooted from their homes, property destroyed and lives wasted and such horrors as Belsen and Buchenwald concentration camps, described so vividly in the newspapers. That took some of the gloss off it.

At school we soon began to see changes; men were coming back from the war and now out of uniform for the first time in years, and some of these people became school teachers. They had a different perspective on life and wanted to make changes. They had a different attitude having seen life in the raw, and we would sometimes manage to get them off their subjects and tell us of their experiences! These men had learned the art of discipline in a hard school and knew how far to go in dealing with us, but we did not dare to try to be clever; they'd seen it all before and woe betide you if you thought they were a soft touch!

By now at last I was beginning to enjoy some of the work we had to do, apart from mathematics which has remained a problem to me to this day, but I revelled in English literature and history and found the subject of geography made me want to travel. French I found reasonably easy; I obviously did not get to the heart of the matter with the language when some few years later when in France I asked for something in a shop, and the assistant replied in English! Woodwork was looked forward to on a Friday afternoon, and at this I excelled, and still like messing about with bits of wood and finding answers to household problems whenever necessary.

But life was not all school; we flirted with paper rounds, but this necessitated a very early start and was rapidly abandoned, and for a while I went out on Saturdays with the baker's rounds man, Mr Evans in his electric van, taking the bread to customers. With a name like that he had to be a Welshman, and would sing as he went from call to call. For this work I earned the princely sum of half a crown, which, added to my pocket money of one shilling per week, made me feel reasonably affluent.

As men were coming back from the war, one of these young men, I doubt if he was more than twenty-eight, returned to the town, and with his parents attended our chapel. My parents knew his family well, and soon learned that Alan had ambitions of going into business, and he subsequently bought a small run-down cycle shop in the town with his army gratuity, and after a few weeks looked for a part-time assistant to help with the repairs, which in those straightened times were numerous, because everybody but the very well-off used bicycles for transport and there was a great shortage of bits and pieces for cycles. So many were in poor condition because of the war, and needed attention. Rubber for tyres was in short supply like everything else, so tyres ran thin and frequently punctured, and he employed me to help with repairs at which I became quite expert, and learned to make up wheels with the spokes all in the right order, change worn out brake blocks and so on after school and all day Saturday.

After a time, as the business progressed. More advanced gadgets were in the pipe line, such as little motors with a small 50 cc petrol engine that was either attached to the back wheel, or was included at manufacture within the wheel itself. These caused a lot of interest as they gave people more mobility and were not all that expensive, and as more were sold nationally, so the prices gradually fell. But owners' clubs developed, and owners did all kinds of modifications to make them go faster! One customer that I can remember was a Mr Fairy, not exactly an intellectual giant, but a good old Hertfordshire peasant who worked on a local farm.

He was in the shop one Saturday enthusing over his acquisition, which he had painted in bright colours. It was parked against the curb outside the shop and a small crowd of kids were round it and laughing at the colours, he heard their comments and went rushing out and shouted at these Philistines, 'Clear orf you lot, that's moine, not yourn!'

This caused a lot of amusement to these kids who fell about laughing. It became a catchphrase which we used frequently thereafter, reducing us all to giggles.

I stayed with Alan until I left school and learned a lot from him, not only about cycle maintenance, but about life in general. He was a serious Christian man who had seen life on active service in the jungle war in Burma and had some idea what made humans tick and what mattered in life; not the sort of propaganda I was used to, and it put a lot of what had been rammed into me into perspective, and taught me to laugh, or ignore, some of the more fanciful ideas that were current in the fundamentalist movement. I treasure his memory as one who made an impact on my life for good.

He was also a very generous man, and after I had been with him for two years he suggested that it was time he had a holiday, he was thinking of going to Switzerland, and asked if I would like to go with him.

This was beyond my wildest dreams; I would pay for the accommodation, the rest he would pay for.

So we went, much to the envy of my friends, and had a wonderful time. By train as well! What a thing to happen to me, a kid from a housing estate in 1947!

5

LIFE GETS SERIOUS

All was not well on the family front. My father became seriously ill, and after much investigation of his condition he was taken to hospital for surgery, which proved to be a disaster, and he was sent home to die.

We had all been doing so well as a family. Both my brothers were progressing well in their lives, and things looked set well for my future, with the school certificate on the horizon, in which I had been told I had a good chance of getting satisfactory grades.

My immediate cry of course was 'why does this have to happen to us?' with the usual selfishness of the young. The next three months for the whole family was a dreadful time. Everybody who knew us from relatives to neighbours were, or seemed to be, involved in helping us. The chapel pulled out all the stops, and much and many prayers were said for my poor father, mother and we three boys. My father suffered terribly with his condition, and as we watched him quickly slip away from this world he changed into a dying man, and my mother suffered with him. However, we were childish enough to still go out and kick a football around, but that is what the insouciance of the young one does at that age!

However the day came that Father passed away, we had all the sympathy you could imagine, but I was now without a father. The church had prayed for his healing; it never struck me at that time why we should expect a miracle to happen, why for us? The answer was of course, why not? What's so special that we should be singled out by the Almighty for preferential treatment when others who did not have our beliefs would not get the same benefits? But eventually I did come to see that miracles rarely happen as we want or expect them to, but our beliefs did give us the miracle of knowing that we had to go on and would find comfort and support from the friends who loved us.

The funeral was held some days later at the chapel. The place was packed as all his many friends and colleagues and just about all of our relatives came to swell the numbers. The funeral service was a celebration of Dad's life; he had been a faithful soul to the chapel and all its affairs, and in his belief in the goodness of God, who'd seen him along with many others during the war through difficult times, and believed that it would all work out in the end, as he used to say, 'for the best'.

With all the organisation it was quite an exciting time for me, but much comfort was afforded to my mother and we his children by the kindness and help from all those people who knew us. I found the interment strangely troublesome however, the minister referring to Dad by his Christian name, a thing this rather magisterial man had never done before.

We were all emotionally exhausted at the end of the day, and it was weeks before my mother smiled again. We continued to attend the chapel weekly, but it was sometime before I could get it out of my head that we'd been unfairly treated by the Almighty, little realising with the ignorance of youth that the only things in life that were inevitable were death and taxation!

It was a long time before I came to appreciate the fact that we had all been brought together by this tragedy and had found our comfort in each other. I now had to find answers to my future; could my poor mother allow me to continue at school? She could not in all reality keep me and younger brother housed fed and watered with no income. My elder brother by now had left school and was training to be a dental technician, but she had only a pittance from her widow's pension, which was not enough to keep us all. However she went to see the headmaster of my school for advice; he was helpful and persuaded her to let me stay on, but she would need to go out to work, which she did, and the headmaster did all he could to find me a congenial training post. I didn't really know what I wanted apart from something to do with railways. He found a course that he thought would suit me at the LMS works at Rugby as an apprentice railway engineer, but after a lot of thought Mother decided she could not bear the thought of my going away from home at this time, so I did not accept. I did stay on and get my school certificate, stayed working with Alan, who had been a tower of strength to me through this time, and looked around for something else to do.

Whilst my father had been in hospital I had met a school friend of mine who was working at the hospital as a student nurse. I met him again after my father had died, and we were talking about the problems of losing a parent, and he told me of one or two patients he had known who had had the same problem as my father. He told me of the work that went into diagnosis and treatments, and his part in it as a nurse. This sounded very interesting to me; I had always been interested in human biology at school in science lessons, and having spent so much time in hospital in my early days, at one time I wanted to study medicine, so I made enquiries, went for an interview with the matron at the hospital, and on 9th November 1949 started as a student at the Lister Hospital Hitchin for the profession which has lead me to the most fulfilling thing I could have done with my life, and as I look back, this was the miracle I needed and never expected. Prayers are always answered, but not necessarily the way you want them to be! My father's death led to a lot of lives being changed by my actions.

6

THE REAL WORLD

The Lister Hospital was a medium sized country town hospital, which at that time had a well-earned reputation for excellence. It was a general hospital and started life before the war as an 'emergency' hospital, one of many built by the government knowing that war was coming. Care and treatment centres needed to be spread around the land, away from the big cities which were vulnerable to aerial bombing in the event of hostilities.

It was built in the grounds of the old workhouse, and as was common in those days the workhouse was renamed the Lister Hospital to make it more respectable, but it remained much the same, with rows of elderly patients confined to their beds and waiting to shuffle off this mortal coil; geriatric care had a lower priority then than it has now! But the acute hospital was built as a series of permanent brick one-storey wards, and then as war seemed imminent, continued with wooden temporary ones which remained until the sixties, I believe, when the whole lot closed down and moved to a brand new purpose-built hospital up the road in Stevenage.

However it was the attitude of the staff that mattered, and it had a good reputation and a nice working atmosphere. There were some 250 nursing staff; half of these were student nurses in training and were looked after by the matron, a regal figure, and her two assistants, the 'ass mat' as we knew her, the home sister and the nurse tutor. These were aided in their care by a very basic physiotherapy department, with one physiotherapist, a pharmacist with a porter, and the hospital porters and ground staff under a fearsome Mr Brown as head porter, who you did not upset if you valued your life, a kitchen to serve staff and patients, and a dietician.

The laboratory was basic in those days but seemed to be adequate. The medical staff consisted of the medical director who was also the senior general surgeon, two registrars, two housemen, and an anaesthetist. On the medical side was a senior physician, two registrars and two house men. These were implemented by visiting consultants from various hospitals, some from London, some from other small hospitals in the area, and a consultant in charge of the lab – all in all for a small town just about enough to be going on with.

As far as I was concerned as a student, the person I was responsible to was the nurse tutor, a lady whose idea of teaching was to read out great chunks from a textbook for us to write down. After a time I got wise to this and found a copy of this textbook and so no longer needed to waste so much ink! I found this attempt at educating us rather ad hoc, and used as I was to professional teachers at grammar school, I was rather disappointed.

We started in our small group of some ten people, a very mixed-ability group I recall. I was the only one with any form of secondary education, and apart from the lectures that we had to attend in our own time which were given by various doctors, press ganged into doing it (and it showed!), it was all a bit of a mystery to most of us. I was fortunate; having been a patient, I had some knowledge of what the nursing profession was about, but most of the others in the group had as much an idea of what they had let themselves in for as studying Greek. After a month of listening to all the reading of lessons, working late in lectures on anatomy and physiology by doctors who did not know how to teach, and talks on simple hygiene, the nurse tutor left, and was replaced by a proper tutor who had studied at university and knew what we as students needed. Life then was demystified, and we were able to question and take part in the process of learning, which made all the difference. We later learned that the previous tutor was not qualified to teach, and was a stop gap until Mr Chapman, the new man, was appointed.

We were in our initial block of study, as it was called, for three months, in which we were taught the rudiments of caring for the sick. Again I was fortunate in that I already knew something about nursing care. I had suffered some appalling treatment from unqualified staff as a patient, but had also had some wonderful care from nurses who really understood my predicament. Three months' stay in an acute ward taught you who to trust and what was needed for your comfort.

Unfortunately all the teaching for us was in the classroom, and practice including bed bathing, giving enemas, injections and simple dressings on a plastic dummy did not really equate with reality; plastic dummies don't respond to pain, or complain if the staff are a bit rushed and skimp care, or complain when they are not covered properly and get cold. Bed making was easy in the classroom, but dirty incontinent patients who needed sheets changing were a different experience and one's olfactory nerves got a bit of a battering!

So after an exam at the end of this introductory block, those of us who passed, and I cannot recall anyone who failed, were allocated to our first ward, and with great trepidation had to face patients who thought we knew what we were doing! After all, we were nurses and wore the uniform, and most patients in hospital were as apprehensive as we were anyway.

My first foray into the wards was a bit of a disaster. I didn't know what to expect. One of my first tasks was to empty a patient's urine bottle which was full of heavily blood-stained and infected urine, which had a smell like I had never met before – once smelt, never forgotten! He'd had an operation on his bladder and a tube was draining the urine into another bottle tied by a length of bandage to the side of the bed. No fancy plastic drainage bags as found nowadays! But as I untied the bottle to empty it into the bucket, it slipped through my fingers and upended and drained into my right shoe, much to the amusement of the patient who said, "Don't worry lad, it'll make you grow!"

The rest of the shift I had to work without socks. It took about a month before the smell faded from the shoes. I certainly could not afford another pair and just had to suffer and leave them outside at night!

We were moved from ward to ward at some two-month allocations, and learned to cope with the myriad problems of what was then modern medicine; looking at it from all these years later, it was pretty basic stuff and at times quite crude. However, we learned, not because we were taught, but when something we did not understand was put before us, we were told by the ward sister or the staff nurse to go with so and so and watch what they did! The concept was basically 'sitting with Nellie', the old apprentice idea, and gave little idea of what was required; you just learned that by default! You ended up knowing what to do, but not why, or when, or when not to do it! This of course was training, not education!

Priorities were not often mentioned; the task had to be done, so get on with it. I recall one day dropping a pint glass bottle of blood which smashed to pieces as it hit the floor as it was about to be transfused into a seriously ill patient, and being well and truly bawled out for making such a mess! It didn't seem to matter about the waste of blood!

We had to clear up messes anyway. There were no cleaning teams at all; each ward kitchen had a ward maid who kept that clean and provided coffee for the ward sister and consultants. That appeared to be, in this very hierarchical society, their main preoccupation. The first hour of every day was spent in pulling the beds away from the wall and sweeping and then polishing the floor with what were called bumpers. This was then followed by bed making – why in this order I will never know, as the blankets filled the ward with dust anyway. It's a wonder infection was not more rife than it was; maybe as personal hygiene was less considered a priority in life in those days, everybody had a better resistance to bugs than in this age of antibiotics.

So we moved from medicine to surgery to the children's ward, the operating theatre and the out patients department, and gleaned a smattering of knowledge from each, interspersed with a fortnight to a month in class every few weeks, where fortunately we could bleed all over Mr Chapman, thank heaven for that man! He did manage to put it in perspective for most of us, but as we hit the floor running there was little time to think, as ever in hospital life the work never stopped. But we were happy in the job; there was so much to see and to be involved in. At the end of this first year we were to be entered for the mock preliminary state examination which consisted of three written papers and a viva, or practical as it was known. Fail to pass this and you would be given a chance to resit it, and if you failed again you were dismissed. So the exam came and went, and I failed miserably. I was torn off a strip by the tutor, told to pull my socks up, I was assured that I was quite capable and should be ashamed of myself for my miserable performance, and indeed I was ashamed – it was my own fault. This was told to me in the presence of my colleagues who all thought that with my educational background I would succeed anyway, but I had been lazy and needed a good kick. And it did work; when I resat the exam after a month I achieved a good result and was told in no uncertain terms not to behave like that again, after all I was being paid £10 a month to be there!

The real preliminary state exam followed a month after that and I had to go to Chase Farm Hospital in Essex for this, and after my previously disastrous effort at the mocks, I did succeed and got a good pass.

Then another tutor was appointed to join Mr Chapman. The health service was in its infancy and was set to expand, and instead of the old hospital management committees, the state was taking over, and there was more money available and the educational side was going to have a higher priority than before.

The new tutor was a rather regal lady, and we were told she would be more involved with the female nurses, leaving Mr Chapman to deal with us men as his main priority. This suited us well, because in those days we did not have to work on any of the women's wards, so there was little point in learning about gynaecology, and we could concentrate on male conditions. We only needed a working knowledge of gynaecology, no great detail of the subject.

Also with the advent of the NHS, two of the other local hospitals were going to be amalgamated with us for administrative reasons, so we began to get a new influx of staff, and also as these other hospitals were not closing to patients, we could be allocated to them as our training needs arose. But the education dept now was solely at the Lister and became a lot busier and more interesting.

So at the end of the first year caring for the sick, trying to learn how to care, and survive this, at times, hair-raising life, what had I learned, or at least what had I achieved?

There had been emotional moments, one or two frightening ones when I felt responsible for things when they went wrong, but there were few people to whom you could open your hearts to and talk it through. We had at the time a lot of Irish girls recruited to cover our shortfall of staff; not everyone wanted to be involved in such work as nursing. The social scene had changed; few young women from upper-class families now felt the call to the caring professions, other things were open to them such as university admission, and the type of person entering the profession was different. People like me, for example, would not have been acceptable before the war, which cessation was only four years away in the recent past, and now the NHS looked abroad and anywhere they could to recruit. Ireland at that time was a fruitful field for workers; the Irish girls were strict church goers and insisted that even though the wards would be depleted on a Sunday morning, they had to go to mass, and had the approval of the authorities as an ethnic minority which had to be humoured. But there was one girl, English as it happened, who was a very sincere Catholic but never boasted of it, to whom I did talk sometimes, and I found her to be a tower of strength. This was of course, having been brought up as a fundamentalist, a contradiction in terms, having been taught that only we as genuine Christians were the holders of compassion, and only we could do God's work here on earth. At least that is what I felt, even though I didn't really believe it!

But to my great surprise, I found that those who had no faith at all were people of great kindness and compassion, and cared for the sick with great humility and love. They may not have always expressed their feelings in words, but by their actions as Nicodemus, the Hellenistic lawyer in the New Testament was told, the spirit of God lands on a lot of unsuspecting heads and directs their lives for the good of mankind, even if they don't know it!

In this year I had learned a lot about myself and was beginning to work out my own priorities in life,and, having seen so much death and misery, I was slowly changing from a rather flippant youth into a more serious person, who now questioned much of my previous teachings as uninformed about life, and indeed extremely shallow and ignorant.

7

GETTING TO GRIPS WITH THE JOB

So life began to get serious! I had by now had a modicum of experience in caring for the sick and a lot of knowledge of anatomy and physiology, and it was time to advance to theatre work and night duty where some of the theory I had acquired would be put into practice.

The thought of the operating theatre was rather worrying at first, but having now been taught the rudiments of team work where everyone had a part to play, here there was no room for individualists. I found that I settled quite well after the initial start at the bottom, by learning the use of all the instruments, their maintenance and sterilisation techniques, and also the way they were set out on the trolleys for the surgeons to work from, and for the assisting nurse to hand them over at the correct time in the operation and indeed the correct instrument. Surgeons do not suffer fools gladly and could get very cross if the wrong forceps were put into his hand at the wrong time. However, having learned the art of scrubbing up and being dressed in the correct sterile gown and gloves and feeling very important, one soon felt rather humble when it was your job to take the case, as it was known, or assist, often standing and holding a retractor for sometimes what felt to be ages, and having to resist the temptation of nodding off and leaning on the patient's chest, and getting moaned at by the anaesthetist because you were limiting the patient's respiratory effort. "The patient needs oxygen even if you don't, nurse!" was the usual remark.

However, it did prove to me to be a most interesting allocation, but I was very annoyed to find that at the end of the month, half my salary was deducted for accommodation when I had to sleep at the hospital on call, and complained that I felt it was unfair that I had to pay to work there! The hospital did not see it my way, I was told to put up or shut up. I had volunteered to be a nurse and that was one of the things I'd better get used to in future. The learning curve was steep indeed!

I was living at home and helping the finances on the domestic scene – not that we were very well paid, about £10 a month – but it was rather tiring at times as I had to cycle four miles to work and back at the end of each shift, and on split shifts could ride quite a few miles a day in all kinds of weather. I certainly could not afford the bus fare, and the bus stops both at home and at the hospital were very inconvenient, and it would have meant a long walk both before and after duty. It was also very tiring after a twelve-hour night, and six nights a week to go on like this, but I was young and managed to survive. If I wanted to do this job, then that was the price one paid. Looking back on it now, this was the age when the concept of the teenager did not exist; you left school at either fourteen or sixteen and worked, there were few social benefits, you got out of life only what you put in, and in care of the sick you put your all into what you did.

My first night duty as a junior was working with a senior student who was in charge of the ward for the full shift. The night sister would do her rounds every four hours and keep an eye on us, but to stay awake was sometimes difficult. Not that there was a lot of time to sit down, with wards of thirty-eight beds, and two side wards always full with patients having all kinds of needs, and when the work permitted, the making of dressings, then packing of drums of these dressings for sterilisation, and other physical tasks which today, with the advent of pre-packed equipment do not happen. It kept you at all times on your toes. One did a round, every ten minutes, of the ward; there was always somebody awake, either in pain, or sleepless due to their condition, or worried about something, and needed either a warm drink, or a position change in bed, or a bandage reapplied, or a quiet chat, and so it went on night after night until you got your night off and collapsed into bed and tried to make up the sleep, until it was time to start again for a whole twelve weeks' allocation. I was fortunate in that living at home I could sleep; the house was empty all day and in a quiet part of the town, but for people who lived in the nurses' home it was always busy with nurses coming on and going off duty, and rather noisy. I recall that one Sunday night with Mother and my brothers at chapel I overslept and did not wake up until eight o'clock, then had to hurry down the road to the phone box and find an excuse, but was still expected to go. There was little give in the system, we were always working on a knife's edge for numbers of staff, and if one person was off for any reason it was difficult to fill the gap. I received a real admonishment for that and never did that again!

The arrangement of care was almost traditional, the patient was of course supposed to be the centre of our attention, but I could never see why the seriously or very ill patients had to be sorted out first irrespective of what else was happening on the ward in the morning; so we started to get them washed and changed and their beds made, often at 4.00 a.m., so that the day staff could get on with the routine business of the day when they came on duty at 8.00 a.m. That was the old tradition of the 'this is what we always do' brigades' attitude and did not change for some years.

One other onerous task each night was to make the porridge for the patients' breakfast for the day staff to serve when they came on duty at 8.00 a.m. This was made from water and raw oat meal and made in a porringer. It needed a special technique to get it right, or it ended up as a solid lump of gloop and had to be thrown out and started again. I never did quite master it, and often got moaned at for the amount I wasted! But it was all part of the day to day, or night to night hassle to get finished by the morning.

So after the first night duty, having learned a lot about staying awake when you desperately wanted to sleep, I assume it was a good discipline, but a hard one for a young teenager to learn! I never enjoyed the experience of night duty in all my years in the profession, and felt that it often prevented me from giving my best.

Now that the hospitals in the area had amalgamated, I was allocated to the small hospital down the road called the North Herts Hospital. This had two wards, both surgical, one for each sex, and a maternity unit which was the province of the midwifery school and nothing to do with us.

They were old-style wards with a large covered balcony at the end of the ward looking out onto the gardens. These were rather pleasant places for convalescent patients to sit during the day and watch the world go by, with a distant view of the main road to Luton. In those far off days we did have convalescent patients, partly because the district nursing services were not so well developed as today, care at home was limited and keeping a patient in bed following an operation was considered essential to give them time to heal, and care at home would have been impossible. I can recall my own experience only some years previously, when after my appendix was removed I was kept in bed for a week post-operatively, and when allowed up could hardly walk, and bed sores were reasonably common due to the lack of exercise for the patient. But things were changing, and we were beginning to realise that the sooner we got our patients back on their feet, the quicker they could go home to a normal life.

I was on duty on one of these wards one night and had a patient with chronic asthma admitted. It was a very hot and sultry night, and although he was receiving oxygen via a facemask, he was very uncomfortable and breathless. I thought it would help the poor old chap if I wheeled him out onto the balcony and covered him up to protect him from anything untoward, to see if this helped. He thought this would be wonderful; he was an outdoor man, a gardener if I remember correctly, and so I wheeled him outside. The night sister when she came to do her rounds was most upset to see an empty space and demanded to know where the patient had got to. I told her why I had done it, you didn't do things like that without permission and she told me off, as she was speaking to me there was a commotion outside on the balcony, it sounded like a couple of shunting engines and she said, "Quick, come on let's see what damage you've caused." We rushed out; the old boy was fast asleep, but a couple of hedgehogs under the balcony were experiencing carnal relations very enthusiastically with maximum noise and enjoyment!

I think that a lot of change occurred because we had an influx of staff from other countries. One year we had a number of South African-trained nurses who sought employment with us to further their careers. I don't really think they did learn a lot from us, as we were thoroughly reactionary, but we did learn a lot from them which proved to be very useful, and did raise a few eyebrows among our rather conservative authorities!

However, I began to enjoy this small hospital work, not quite so busy as the bigger general hospital. I met a young lady with whom I formed a special attachment; it started off on a professional level by discussing work after our initial introduction to each other, but soon developed into a deep friendship in which eventually we fell in love, and life took on a different perspective from then on. The problem was we were not always able to see each other when we wanted; the allocation people didn't take personal preferences into account, we were allocated according to our stage of training and the requirements of the wards, and if night duty or a move to another hospital occurred we had to put up with it.

Pam was about six months ahead of me in the training schedule and was working in the theatre when we first met. I had gone to the theatre to bring a patient back to the ward following surgery to his hand and fingers which had been cut badly in a building site accident. As the patient was wheeled out of the anaesthetic room by this rather good-looking and willowy young lady, she was very excited and said to me, "Dr Forbes, let me sew these wounds up on my own." I was somewhat taken aback by this remark as we were not allowed to participate in treatment, only care, and I said, "Bet they all get infected then and his fingers drop off with gangrene!" Most ungallant, but that was our first meeting, and she did frequently remind me of my remark! I don't recall ever apologising either, even after we were married some years later!

Life with its many facets continued. It was nearly Christmas and preparations were being made for the festivities on the wards. They were great fun, very democratic for a few days, even the matron showed her human face, and to see the senior surgeon operating on the turkey at Christmas dinner was a sight worth seeing, dressed up in theatre gown and gloves assisted by the head porter, the much-feared Mr Brown.

Yes, hospital life was fun for all its misery and trauma for the patients at times, but often the funny side was seen. If you didn't laugh sometimes you would need to cry, but you learned not to let your feelings show too much.

I had now passed into my third year and was classed as a senior student, and had to take charge of a ward at night with a junior nurse to assist me. This was a bit daunting at first but you soon got used to the responsibility. We were well-trained, and as I look back on those three years I realise how much I'd changed over that time, and was now judged competent, or we would not have been allowed to do what we did, and on reflection, I realise now that in spite of poor teaching, by hitting the ground running, we learned to survive – had we not done so, we would have done a lot of damage and been in serious trouble.

The final exam was to be taken in May 1953. This exam was held at the Wittington Hospital in London. I had been told that I could stay at the Lister Hospital if I passed the exam until I left to do my National Service the following January, but would have to be on permanent nights until that time. This was not a pleasing prospect, but it was customary for nurses when they qualified to leave and seek a post at other hospitals. So I was lucky that this rule was waived for me, and when I qualified in the July, and with great pride wore the epaulettes on my shoulder pads with the silver letters SRN thereon, and like many others before me began to find that I still had much to learn, I had in reality only just scraped the surface!

I'd had my twenty-first birthday party in June of that year and most of my family and Pam and her parents attended. A good time was had by all, apart from the many warnings handed out to me in speeches by those fundamentalist relatives present about the snags and pitfalls I would encounter in life as I joined the services for my National Service. Some of these po-faced uncles and aunts failed to appreciate that I had seen too much already of the results of the seamy sides of life when caring for the sick, and the experiences I'd had had made me well aware of what could happen if one did not base one's life on a firm ethic. They would not have been very keen to have known however that Pam and I planned in the following September to go on holiday together to stay at a hotel in Bournemouth, and would have been shocked at this flagrant social gaffe as they would see it, even though we had separate rooms at the hotel!

The next few months passed quickly, Christmas 1953 came and went and it was time for me to put off my civilian uniform, and join the ranks of the RAF for what I could not foresee then, indeed or wanted to at the time, to be my home for the next twenty-two years, until I rejoined the NHS in 1977.

POSTSCRIPT TO PART ONE

So this was the first part of my journey through life. It was partaken in the main in the company of many good and loving people, and my wonderful parents in particular, indeed all 'pilgrims going to a better land'.

The second part I recount in my previous book *To Travel Hopefully* which tells of my life in the RAF medical branch, until I was employed once again by the NHS. Many, if not most, of the people that I have mentioned have completed their journeys and arrived at their better land. We have no knowledge of what the land was that they found when they arrived, but most, if not all, travelled hopefully, and as they got older and wiser, found that along with countless others, and as I did, the greatest pleasure and satisfaction in life was in helping others less fortunate than themselves along those thorny paths. The second part of this narrative deals with my life as I leave the RAF and return to the NHS, and finally as a qualified acupuncturist build my own private practice, which in turn developed into a limited company, and in this I had to use all the skills and expertise I had learned in my previous life to achieve what I was trying to do. 'To cure sometimes, to relieve often, but to comfort always'.

I think that this last part of the story was without doubt where it all came together and I was doing what I really wanted to do, and doing it my way for all the right reasons! But then, the best laid plans of mice and men…

End of Part One

To the memory of my dearest Pam who left this life in May 2006.

PART TWO

Nurse Education and Alternative Medicine
(Life from both sides of the divide)

PROLOGUE

My last few days in the RAF at the end of twenty-two years' service, and recently in charge of the nurse training school at the RAF hospital Ely, were passing quickly. My demobilisation date was June 3rd 1977 and I was looking forward to a change of lifestyle as I became a civilian again, but did not think that I would inadvertently almost bankrupt myself before I began! Had it not been for an honest car salesman I nearly did!

My application for the post of tutor in charge of pupil nurse training at The District Hospital in Peterborough had been accepted. The then-director of nurse education advertised the post and, as he told me on the phone, he wanted somebody to take the pupil nurse training off his hands as he had more than enough to do with training the student nurses.

It was agreed at interview that I would spend a few days of my terminal leave experiencing life at the new school of nursing, and I realised at once that my old car would not take kindly to a journey of some sixty miles a day, so I gave it to my teenage son – who was delighted with it and covered it with go faster tape and other useless goodies – and negotiated the purchase of a new one from the main dealer, and paid for it out of my terminal gratuity.

So I bought my first new car – and what a thrill it was, red, gleaming and very small, and mine! I couldn't afford a bigger one but it felt like a Rolls to me! As my wife Pam and I sat in the car showroom, I prepared to write what was for me up to that time the biggest cheque I'd ever written, for £2300, an immense sum for me at that time in 1977, but the average price of a new small car in those days.

The salesman turned to Pam who was talking and said, "Wait a minute, or your husband will make a mistake."

I handed the cheque to him, he looked at it and laughed, "See what I mean, have you got that amount of money?" he asked her. I'd written £23,000. A hasty rewrite amended this gaffe!

We were driven down to the new car compound in the company's staff car, a top of the range model, and as we relaxed in the luxurious leather seats and glided along in comfort, I turned to Pam and said, "We'll get one of these one day."

She laughed and replied, "That'll be the day!"

But one day in the distant future, many years down the line, the day arrived and we did get one, and a lot of other goodies, but that was not going to happen on the salary of a teacher of nursing in the NHS as you will see!

1

NEW BEGINNINGS

Suddenly it was May 13th 1977, the last day of my service in the RAF, and the start of my month's terminal leave, and I have to admit to my shame that by eleven o'clock a.m, I was filthy stinking drunk! It wasn't my fault. "Oh really!" I hear you say. "A man in your position of trust, and you expect us as intelligent readers to believe that?"

But no, it really wasn't my fault, let me explain as I try to recover my good name! Are you sitting comfortably? Well, here we go!

My departure was interrupted by many telephone calls of best wishes, and by 1100 hours I was having a cup of coffee before my last lecture to a group of nurses, which hopefully would conclude at midday. I would then hand in my uniform, and documents, and book myself out of the mess, to rejoin civilian life.

Another nursing colleague arrived in a hurry with a large bottle of sherry for myself and my staff to have a celebratory farewell drink, we found an assortment of glasses and cups to partake of this valedictory swill, but on attempting to open the bottle, she dropped it on the stone floor of the office where it broke into 1000 pieces! Some omen for the future I thought!

Amid much banter and laughter, we managed to mop up the sherry with some paper towels. It was a very warm day and unfortunately by the time we'd mopped it up, the fumes had risen from the floor, and unrealised by us all, we had inhaled a considerable quantity of alcohol and we were now quite drunk!

If I recall correctly, and with some difficulty, I assume that my blood alcohol level was well above the permitted level for driving, farewells were said and a lot of emotion expended. Why is it when you are drunk, friends become very good friends and you are reluctant to part from them?

However, I pulled myself together as best I could, wiped the tears from my eyes and went into the classroom of waiting students. If I remember correctly, and with some difficulty, to deliver my last lecture, on the rather sombre subject of care of the dying both physically and emotionally, which I was told later caused more laughter than the latest Goon Show! I then had to be lead gently from the classroom and advised to sit down!

I do hope that somebody on the staff eventually gave them the correct version of that lecture!

So for me that was the end of an era. I went out not so much with a bang, but with a drunken whimper!

So a fortnight later, after a short break, it was time for me to return to the NHS which I had left in 1954 and attempt to fit myself back into civilian life.

The director of education at my new hospital was off sick on my arrival, and his deputy Jack was in charge of affairs. Jack was a very experienced man, a quiet and reflective chap who knew his job inside out, and I found that he was a colleague one could turn to for advice, and he proved to be a friend who was willing to help at all times.

The other tutorial staff were women of various ages. I was used to working in a female-dominated profession, but these were not like their equivalents in the RAF, being people who had worked their way up the ladder in the same hospital and were therefore rather parochial in their beliefs and actions.

There was one other person, most important, she knew everything that went on: the school secretary. One to cultivate and not to upset if I wanted to survive in that setting!

First impressions to me were that it was a rather reactionary and very conservative set up, and coming from a service where there was a lot of movement of staff bringing in new ideas and practices, to me it proved to be rather stultifying. Most of the ladies in the department were of the old school and only knew life in the local hospital.

We had weekly meetings to 'discuss matters' in principle, but the day was usually carried by the director when he eventually returned to duty. He was a nice man and purported to be a democratic leader – always leading from the front, but it was he and he alone that allowed anything new to be brought in to the day's work.

Little innovation was possible in that sort of set up; it was looked upon as disruptive, disturbing the even tenure of their ways.

New Beginnings

One of my surprises was the inefficient way the training records of the nurses was held. This was of course before the advent of the easy-to-use computer systems of today, but when I wanted to find individual records I had to trawl through masses of ledgers to find what I wanted.

The nurse's details were all in great tomes, each intake in its own book, not in alphabetical order but just as they came. The only reference to make it easier was the date of intake – little help with some 250 nurses on the books, all in different stages of training. To compliment these details each nurse had a separate file, again kept in the same way, and to delve through this lot was quite daunting. Cross referencing appeared to be unknown.

I asked if this was not too time-consuming to find anything in a hurry, and was told that this was the way it had always been done and they were quite used to it, and I'd soon catch on! I asked if they'd heard of the Kardex visible edge recording system; I was obviously talking a foreign language, no they hadn't and were happy with this as it was!

One day sorting out rubbish – and there was plenty of it in my new office – I found a large box at the back of a cupboard, it was full of a brand new Kardex system, still in its cellophane wrappers! I showed it to the secretary who said she'd seen it but didn't know what it was for, so she put it in the cupboard out of the way! When I explained to her how it worked, she replied that it wouldn't work here as we had too many staff, so I went to work on it myself, giving each nurse I was responsible for a card with a reference number corresponding to the same number I had given to each nurse in the ledger, and filed it all in its Kardex flip folder. Unfortunately, this all had to be done in longhand as the office 'didn't have the time to do that sort of thing'!

A few days later it proved its worth when the director asked me to get the folder for an individual nurse he wanted to dismiss. I immediately went to my Kardex, found the notes, took them back to him and put them on his desk. "What are these?" he said.

"The folder you wanted," I replied.

"But I've only just asked you for them, it usually takes a while to get them." I explained, and so we got the Kardex system, which was not replaced for some years until the computer took over! But by the standards of the day, it was a good school and produced a well-qualified and rounded – in skills terms – product.

A weekly discussion was held in the boss's office when problems were aired. On one of these sessions the behaviour of a particular student was brought up. The conversation turned to semantics, how to describe what she'd done in polite terminology!

I observed that it could be difficult, particularly if the lawyers were involved in her case, and we could find ourselves in trouble, and explained by telling them a rather risqué tale of a problem I encountered once when getting the words wrong. There was a shocked hush and the conversation rapidly turned to other matters; two of the younger tutors present were by now rolling on the floor, which earned them a severe look from the boss!

I was taken aside later by one of the older ladies in the department and informed that the boss was not amused by that sort of humour and didn't want to hear that sort of thing in his school of nursing, at which I laughed loudly, and told her to tell him to come and tell me then, much to the consternation of the messenger!

There were going to be some changes here, I thought. I wasn't taking that and it was an infantile response. When some time later he went off sick, helping to empty his desk drawers, I found a copy of *Playboy* in them, I then realised it was not genuine wrath but just part of the act. He was a very nice man really, as I said! But sadly he became seriously ill and died. Jack took over, and we settled down under his benevolent tutelage and began to enjoy life to the full.

The new extension to the school had just been completed and we moved in at last. It was now a more than adequate education centre, with new offices and classrooms, and we could get on the job with more room and facilities. It also had a large common room which was most useful for socialising. We had more and more visitors to the school as we took on more subjects to teach.

My responsibility was, of course, mainly to the pupil nurses, although I was asked at times to do recruiting sessions at schools and at local sixth form centres in the town, which were a bit of a drag.

We had four intakes a year of some twenty-five pupils, each intake needing a six-week introductory block in class, and five one-week blocks over the next two years.

From the start I was determined to make the learning process more ward-based and, with a certain amount of resistance from my colleagues, started to teach the nurses practical skills on the ward with real patients, instead of plastic dummies in the classroom, under the supervision of the tutorial staff. This had the approval of the ward staff, who could now see that we did know how to do it!

However, I did not want to train nurses, as it was known, but to educate them, and with their knowledge to be able to apply it using their own initiative when necessary if what they found in reality did not always accord with what we had taught them. After all, I've never yet found a sick patient who responded as described in the books!

But many of the routine tasks were standardised in a 'procedure book'. This outlined the basic requirements for numerous onerous tasks such as taking blood pressure, doing a simple dressing or an intramuscular injection, but it was only a guide, and flexibility was needed when doing these tasks, all to be done under supervision of qualified nurses. The trouble was that some staff thought of it as the gospel to be obeyed implicitly.

However, as found in all situations, corners were cut and sometimes things were done in a hurry, which was dangerous, and once or twice I had to take a pupil to task for doing something rather dodgy, to be told that 'this is the way it's done on this ward', which caused a certain amount of acrimony when the information was conveyed to the ward sister. But patient safety was paramount and qualified nurses are responsible by law to do the job properly. A lot of these staff had been in post for years and resented this type of interference in what they saw as their province, but being qualified they could not hide behind 'that's what's always been done here!'

As is usual with people with a lot of experience, change did not come easily, and rarely up to now had they seen tutorial staff on the wards, and this was a great challenge to them.

Because we now had a larger school building we were taking on more students and so needed more tutorial staff, and at last had an infusion of new blood with new ideas and experiences from other hospitals, so I was making more friends to my ideas, and more allies.

Rote learning for me had never been acceptable; I hoped to produce an independent-minded and thinking nurse who would be able to cope with the many problems and changes the profession was going to meet in the future, both educationally and indeed morally. The world was changing rapidly and we needed to keep up with the change, and not just change for the sake of change. We had a lot of thinking to do if we were to progress.

It was an interesting time, and as we took on more staff we became a more democratic organisation. There were more people with more ideas, and they demanded a say in the set up, and some of these people were very clever indeed and were worth listening to.

We now began to enjoy a number of social occasions which would have been unthinkable in the previous regime. We instituted the occasional lunchtime BBQ and various people would come from other departments and chat to us. The Christmas dinner, where everybody did a bit of the preparation at home and it all came together on the day, was well-received and attended by some of the senior officers of the hospital. As you would expect, all tried to excel at the cooking, and a very good meal it was too. A postprandial entertainment was performed by various members of the school staff, again doing their very best in the presence of their colleagues.

The students, of course, had their own social functions (not quite so circumspect as ours!) most of which had to be organised in their own time so that it did not interfere with their studies. There appeared to be developing a very happy atmosphere in the hospital and I felt that this could only be good for patient care. Many years previously, a mental nurse I knew told me of his boss at his first hospital who said, "Contented staff, contented patients."

By and large we were now producing good, caring nurses, and the ward staff commented on this fact frequently to our great pleasure.

I had now been in post for eighteen months and felt that I had found a very comfortable niche in life, working hard, producing excellent nurses and getting good exam results from the pupils. However, we had been without a director now for some time. Jack was first class but had not got the clout of a fully paid up director of education and really major change was a slow progress. We needed a player at the centre of things to represent us, and eventually a new boss was appointed, a very experienced and progressive lady who knew her ways around the corridors of power, and we hoped would make some changes to some of those things we knew needed doing, but up to now we were unable to get them done.

2

UNDER NEW LEADERSHIP

On appointment, the new director was wise enough to leave things alone for some six months and looked at the overall scene. She made a number of minor changes immediately, and of course came across some resistance, but was a persuasive person who usually was able to get her own way. She was certainly not afraid to use and to draw on our own experience and expertise to get things going. I felt she was reasonably open-minded so one day, with some misgivings, I invited one of the local clergy who had, I was told, perfected the art of spiritual healing, to talk to us as a group in the school. Surprisingly she was most interested and promised to be at the meeting.

I had been dipping my toe in the water of alternative medicine for some time. I'd always found the subject interesting having seen the results of acupuncture whilst serving in the Far East, but by and large at this time, most of these therapies were classified as, if not dangerous, diverting people away from 'proper medicine'. But I felt there were possibilities in this we could use. This invitation had come about by chance.

I had a mature pupil nurse on one of my courses who had experienced more than her share of troubles in life, in her marriage, family relationships, health and so on, and now after six months into her course was finding that her health was taking the strain, with heavy lifting, night duty, and running a home becoming too much to cope with.

She was worried that she would not be able to continue with her course, and one afternoon asked me if she could go off early, she had an appointment to see somebody about her back ache. "It's getting worse," she said, "I just can't go on, I've got to do something about it."

"Who's your doctor?" I asked.

She looked a little shame faced, "Not seeing a doctor, I'm going to see a faith healer at a local parish church," she replied and asked, "do you mind?"

"Why should I, there's more things in heaven and Earth…" I quoted. "Let me know how you get on."

She looked relieved at my acceptance of her proposal and limped out of the office. The next morning she came into class on time, walking on air and looking so different from the woebegone figure of the day before who I had seen limping along.

"You look better, what happened?" I asked.

She told me that she had arrived at the church just before four o'clock and the vicar was waiting for her, but she was suddenly overcome with doubt and couldn't accept his invitation to go into the church with him.

"It's alright for you, you go to church, I don't and I felt a bit of a cheat," she said to me.

"What did the vicar say?" I asked, ignoring this last remark.

"He said, well I'm going in, so if you want to come in I'll be waiting for you in the chancel."

She waited about ten minutes, then plucked up courage and sidled into the church very apprehensively to find the vicar sitting at his desk in the chancel. He took her hand, led up to the sanctuary and asked her to kneel at the altar rail.

"It was very quiet in there," she said, "I could hear the traffic outside and the birds singing and I felt I shouldn't be here, but he stood over me, put his hands gently on my head and started to talk very quietly."

"What did he say?" I asked.

"I don't know," she replied, "it was as if he was talking to a friend. Suddenly all my cares and worries went, I stood up, no pain and here I am pain-free."

"I'm going to talk to this man," I said. "What you've told me is very interesting."

I found him the following day at his vicarage: a short, tubby elderly man with a shock of grey hair. He greeted me warmly, we talked of this and that for a few minutes then he told me about himself. He was of Lebanese origin, and during the British mandate in Palestine had been vicar of a well known biblical town, where he discovered he had what he called 'healing hands', and when he came to the UK at the end of the war he continued his work with the sick.

"Would you come and talk to the tutorial staff at the hospital?" I asked him.

"Yes, if you will come to one of my healing services," he replied quickly. So the deal was struck, and next week he came. He proved to be a most able speaker as one would expect him to be, and very lucidly explained to us just what he attempted to do without resorting to evangelical type jargon which is guaranteed to put off most non-churchgoing audiences. Our new director, who claimed to be a sceptic, was impressed, remarking to me afterwards thoughtfully, "That's a man I could talk to."

So one evening a few weeks later my colleague Sophie and I went along to his church not knowing what to expect. It was a lovely summer evening. Local churches are all built of cream-coloured stone and this one was the same as other country churches in this area. It had a particularly fine spire which seemed to go up and up into the deep blue sky on that lovely cloudless evening. As we entered the church I was surprised to find that we were to partake in an ordinary Anglican Eucharist. It was quiet and we found a pew and sat down, the only sound was a single bell calling the faithful to prayer. There were not many present in the congregation and at first I paid little attention to them, just looking forward to enjoying the show!

The service started and worked its way through what was to me the well-known Liturgy. I was expecting something different, and I looked quizzically at Sophie who just shrugged her shoulders.

Just before the Communion, the vicar asked that those in the congregation who would like the 'laying on of hands' after they had taken their Communion, to stay kneeling at the altar rail.

I went up to the rail and made my Communion and returned to my pew, but four people stayed there. The vicar spent about five minutes with each, he placed his hands on their heads and talked very quietly, I was unable to hear what he said it was so quiet, only the murmur of the priest's voice, the soft sound of traffic on the main road outside, and the sound of birds singing.

The four people eventually returned to their pews, there was a charged atmosphere in the church and the sound of somebody softly crying.

The vicar and his deacon then came down into the nave and knelt down, and after a pause said, "Let us pray, let us pray for those who cannot be with us tonight because of their troubles, for Mrs so-and-so, whose son is on the run from prison, Mr and Mrs who are both homeless since his business crashed, and various other poor souls to whom life had given a fatal blow," and so on. A whole group of people down on their luck with nowhere to turn to for help, lonely and unloved.

I looked at Sophie, she gestured to the members of the congregation, then I looked closer and saw a sorry looking mass of humanity, but they were basking – if that is the word – in the attention of this good man, the atmosphere indeed was electric.

After the closing hymn, we left in a rather reflective mood and next day, I went to see the vicar again.

"Well?" he asked, looking me straight in the eye.

I replied, "You were concentrating all your love and care on those poor people, all the agencies appear to have given up on them."

He smiled. "You've got it, nobody wants them or listens to them, only God."

This brought to mind the words spoken by Ambroise Pare, the great French physician of the eighteenth century: 'A physician's role is to cure sometimes, to relieve often, but to comfort always', and I realised that that was my goal in life for the future: to be, as much as anything, a giver of comfort.

It was difficult to assume this role in the nursing profession at that time. Senior nurses still laboured under the mistaken impression that to stand and listen to the patient was wasting time, there was so much more to do in a day's work. I was struck as I developed my skills, particularly when in private practice, just how little I had listened in the past, and how much I could have helped had I done so by listening for the clues and sharing with the patient his problems – sharing, the true meaning of the word sympathy! Not empathy, which is just being aware of his problems.

However, this is not just about the difficulties in nurse training, but my role in it now. I was of course still missing my RAF uniform, and found it difficult at times as it was not always obvious just who I was, another figure in a grey suit. Often it involved explaining time and time again to staff in the hospital and telling them my role. In an identifiable uniform in the services your role was obvious, but handling civilian nurses was different. I recall at my teacher training college, a civilian organisation to which I was seconded whilst still serving, we were asked by the director of studies what attitude we expected primarily from our students. I replied, respect, for which sadly I was shot down in flames – you have to earn that, they all said, being very PC!

I argued that every office had a degree of respect to it, that's why you were there, and had proved it by being considered to be a responsible applicant to that office. For example, in the services, the commanding officer might well be a pratt, but he was the boss and was paid to take the can back when it all went pear shaped, but he could soon lose this respect, and it was up to the holder of the office to behave himself. This onslaught was greeted with puzzled silence. So when one's authority, because of sheer disrespect or disobedience, was flouted, one had been able to solve the problem justly and with a lot of thought. Knee-jerk reaction was usually unjust in a free society, and the action taken had to be sufficient to ensure that the culprit learned from their mistake.

One Monday a very street wise young lady announced to me that she would not be attending class one afternoon because she had to take her driving test. I pointed out that her test conflicted with an important visit the class were taking to the operating theatre for a lecture by the nurse in charge, and that she was after all paid by the hospital to work, and not go off on her own affairs in hospital time.

She replied that she had only that day been informed of the test, I pointed out to her she would have had at least a month's notice, as my own daughter had been given ten weeks notice from the same test centre, so no, she could not go with my permission and should arrange another date, and I expected her be at the theatre at two o'clock. At this, she shrugged her shoulders and stormed out of my office, slamming the door behind her.

I went back early from lunch that day, and as I walked up the hospital drive along came a driving school car with this young lady in the driving seat, obviously going to the test!

The rest of the class had gone to their lecture with instructions to be back in class by three o'clock.

On return, the young miscreant was not with them. "Where's Nurse Yelland?" I asked.

"Oh she's around somewhere," they replied evasively.

"Well go and get out of uniform and be back here at four," I told them.

All the nurses arrived back in class at four, including Nurse Yelland. She looked at me rather apprehensively, but I had no intention of confronting her directly and thought I'd play the waiting game. I debriefed the visit, dismissed the class and went to see the director to tell her about the miscreant. She was most indignant and wanted to deal with her straight away.

"Please," I asked, "let me deal with this, she won't do anything like that again and will learn a very hard lesson."

"Alright," she agreed, "but what will you do?"

"Don't worry," I replied, "nothing illegal," and laughed.

So I played the waiting game, and for the rest of the week she appeared to settle down, assuming that she had got away with it.

The last class of the week on Friday, as it was the end of their two years' training, was all about disciplinary procedures, reasons for dismissal and so on and the legal responsibilities of the trained nurse. I also touched on reasons for dismissal and gave a list of crimes which could lose them their position and employment, and one of the reasons was theft, and included not only theft of property, but also theft of time, as in taking time off work but being paid for the time they were not there! Young Nurse Yelland began to sit up and take notice at that and looked a bit sick! I finished at 12.30 p.m., and the afternoon session was to be about form filling for their final exam and for me to give them their last interview before they went off duty. I informed them that the interviews would be in alphabetical order and not as had been the usual practice, where the ones with the furthest to go home were seen first. So Nurse Yelland not only had the farthest to go, but was last in the queue.

The afternoon passed slowly and just before five the miscreant came into my office. She looked rather apprehensive

"Sit down nurse," I said. "Did you pass?"

"Oh yes," she replied smiling, "isn't it wonderful?"

"So you've managed to rescue something from the wreckage of your career, you'd better see me first thing on Monday morning without fail," I replied. "Go on, get out."

She probably had a most uncomfortable weekend, but at nine, on Monday she came in.

"What do you want?" I asked her.

"You said you wanted to see me."

"No I don't, but the director does, so wait here."

The director was in her office. I told her about Friday's interview and the girl's reaction to it. She put down her pen and said, "You'd better send her in."

"No, let her wait, she's on duty, she can come this afternoon before she goes off duty."

"You're a hard man," she said.

"No I'm not," I replied, "she's a member of a profession, she's got to learn, would you like her to walk out on a patient? She is after all being paid to be here, she asked us to train her."

So at 2.30 p.m., she arrived at my office again. "What do you want?" I asked.

"I've got to see the director," she said.

"Not like that," I said, "you know you have to wear uniform when you are seen by her, go and change."

"But I'll miss my bus," she wailed.

"You should have thought of that," I replied unfeelingly. She came back five minutes later in uniform. "Wait here and I'll see if she's free," I told her. I went in to see the boss.

"That girl is here," I said, "but please don't sack her, she's too good to lose."

She was eventually seen at three o'clock. She was in the office for no more than a couple of minutes, but came out very white and shaky! And of course she passed all her exams with flying colours and proved to be a very good member of the nursing team. Hopefully she had learnt a lesson about accountability!

Being solely responsible for some 125 nurses was quite hard work, but very enjoyable. I'd been teaching now for over six years and was settling into a comfortable routine, but the goal posts in the NHS were shifting, and as the workload increased, another staff member was appointed to act as my deputy. Laurie was a widower who had lost his wife recently, and was feeling very lonely and unwanted and needed an interest in life without too much stress. He came from a mining area in the north, and came south to get away from all his memories. He'd been in the RAF, as a nursing attendant, and qualified SRN after his demob.

He was a nice chap, and we hit it off at once and had a happy relationship. He did have a tendency to take over – he was older than I, but not so well qualified – but we worked well together. One thing I always admired about Laurie was his most beautiful copper plate handwriting, so different to my hurried scrawl. He fitted in well, and eventually to our delight married a colleague who was the control of infection officer for the authority. And they made a delightful couple!

It was time to let the springs off and think about summer holidays. Up to this point Pam and I had always arranged family holidays, but our two eldest boys had left home, and our daughter, who was now sixteen, felt she was now far too old to come away with her parents and, with the confidence of the average teenager, volunteered to keep house whilst we were away.

We took a cottage in Snowdonia for a fortnight; in the second week was the marriage of Prince Charles, so we took our colour television with us to see the show, televisions being rare in rented accommodation at that time. I had found this cottage advertised in the AA guide and assumed that as it was expensive it would be a first class rent, and so looked forward to a nice relaxing time in nice surroundings.

One evening my eldest son phoned and told me that he had been promoted to a senior position in his company and would have to move to a different house and neighbourhood as he would be expected to entertain colleagues. Being short of cash in the circumstances he would not be able to afford a holiday that year and both he and his wife needed one! He asked what we were doing that year?

I told him about our proposals. "Lucky old you," he replied, "could we join you?"

Oh dear, what do you say? The outcome of this was that they did join us! Pam was not pleased, she wanted time on our own, she was working as a ward sister in a geriatric hospital and really needed a rest, and didn't speak to me for a couple of days! I should have known better, but had been caught on the hop! But that's family life!

It therefore did not turn out to be the carefree holiday we had expected, but we did enjoyed it even though catering for four meant little rest. But we went up Snowdon and did all the usual tourist things and saw the Prince of Wales' wedding on television. The snag was, however, expensive the cottage may have been, the promise of luxurious accommodation did not materialise!

It was not all lost however, for the first time, under the expert tutelage of my son I learnt how to BBQ properly – up to now my efforts would have been more appropriate to Golders Green Crematorium!

So the holiday came and went, and eventually we packed up for the long journey home. As we trundled along the motorway, we passed some slow moving caravans. I turned to Pam suddenly and said, "That's what we'll get, a caravan! Two berth!"

"Now that's a good idea," she replied. And so began another era in our lives, caravanning.

We arrived home at about 2.00 p.m. and straight away went out to the nearest caravan agent some fifteen miles away, and by 6.00 p.m. were the owners of a top of the range Ace caravan which I collected three days later.

With some trepidation I hitched it up to the car and started for home, and began to experience the delights of getting in the way of all the other traffic! It was a bit hairy, that drive home, fifteen miles had never felt so long, and eventually with a sigh of relief we arrived back and manoeuvred it onto the drive of our house with the intention of going out the next weekend for a stay at the caravan site at Wells-next-the-Sea on the Norfolk coast.

One learns by one's mistakes, and I think we made more than most on our first trip out, but thoroughly enjoyed ourselves. We arrived just as the sun had set, went to bed and awoke to a lovely sunny day, and had our first breakfast on wheels looking out on a brilliant blue sea. This indeed was the life for us!

We had a lot of fun as we learned, and over the years progressed to better and better vans as they developed. Our last one even had central heating, quite an innovation at that time, until I became so busy we had little time for holidays. But by then we had seen more of the country than had many people, and had numerous photographs to bore visitors with if they were interested!

Back at the hospital our new director of education was finding her feet and was making plans for the future.

The General Nursing Council, the training body for nurses, was due to inspect us on its annual visit, the first with our new director. This took place in the early part of 1979 and the inspectors took us apart at the seams.

We were out of date and reactionary, slow to institute new ideas in education and so on, and needed to review the whole of our systems.

We had in reality been using an apprenticeship system which had been alright up to now, but with advances in technology and a change in the expectations of modern students was unacceptable in this day and age, we were told. There were a lot more tools we could use and we needed to accept these, so as to educate our nurses.

Not all these ideas were going to fit the bill, but the liberal thinkers and theorists were having a big say now. To be told that spelling and punctuation was not important when dealing with written work was anathema to me; we were trying to get communication skills high on our list of priorities, and I felt that were the students unable to use their own language correctly, it could well be dangerous to patient care, if they could not report legibly to their seniors and the medical staff in writing, what are or can be in the right circumstances legal documents.

There was also the thinking that all nurses would have the same introductory course and then diversify into other specialties such as mental nursing, midwifery, and so on and getting rid of the SEN, and my role as tutor to the pupils would go under this system, which did not please me. I was just beginning to produce really thoughtful caring nurses, well able to develop their skills in lateral thinking and with good communication skills, and the whole lot was dumped. I protested loudly about this enthusiastic wholesale destruction of a functioning system by ideologues with theories not only untested, but to me out of ignorance of the way the profession worked. I also predicted, accurately as it turned out, that this labour force of learners, which composed at least 50% of the hospital's nursing staff, would need to be filled, and it would be with unqualified and untrained persons from the lower educated classes so they could be paid a lower rate and ostensibly save money, and then I predicted, they would have to appoint agency staff to fill the gap, at vast expense, because unqualified staff could not legally be held to account for bad practice, and the hospital would be caught up in a legal minefield costing thousands. And so it turned out to be!

My protests were in vain, and the clever people and the bean counters won, putting nurses into career and management structures, which took preference over caring for the sick.

The tutorial staff, without any consultation, were directed to new areas. I was sent to the geriatric department to deal with nurses in the clinical situation, completely away from any classroom or administrative control, and as I protested, I was told, 'well leave then, or put up and shut up!' And education on the hoof as it were, in the clinical situation, particularly when dealing with senior staff unable to accept new ideas, was discouraging to say the least.

They had pulled the carpet from under my feet and I was for a time at a loss to know what to do for the future, and unfortunately I had few choices available, unless I chose to go in a different direction, which is what I eventually did.

3

WAKING UP

Things sometimes happen which alter the course of one's life. In spite of the disappointment of finding myself in what I thought was going to be a dead-end post, I was beginning to find pleasure again in dealing with sick people in a hands-on situation, and learnt how to plan my day's work and not be beholden to the ward staff.

Dealing with educational matters on the hoof in a hard-pressed nursing situation was difficult, indeed I still felt a little in the way at times, and then an event occurred which made me feel much more valuable to the ward and helped my rather deflated ego.

A patient called Mrs Newbold was an eighty-nine-year-old lady with a terminal condition, but was surviving rather well with care. However, I was rarely taken into a patient's confidence; most were aware of my role, which was to look after the nurses' educational needs.

One morning I was therefore somewhat surprised to be asked by this well-spoken and obviously intelligent lady if she could talk to me in confidence. She had a potentially fatal condition called aortic aneurysm in which the main artery from the heart was diseased and weakened, and this could burst at any time without warning, causing her instant demise. I pulled the curtains around the bed, sat down and took her hand in mine.

"What's the problem?" I asked.

"I want to die," she replied, "I've had enough, I've outlived my family, my property has been sold, I've no friends, they've all gone, and all I own is in the locker at the side of the bed and the bank. Can you help me to die quickly?"

This was a cry from the heart and could not be ignored; the desperation showed in her face and needed an immediate considered response. I was a little surprised at her request; she was a devout Roman Catholic and I felt this was unusual in somebody with such a faith as she had.

"I can understand what you want Mrs Newbold," I replied slowly, "but I cannot perform any action which would result in your death, but then I don't want you to die." She looked at me curiously.

"Why not?" she asked.

"Well, firstly that would be murder, secondly, we'd have to clear the mess up."

"Thirdly?" she asked, smiling.

"Well you were once a very important person in a lot of persons' lives, a mum, a company secretary I believe, and there were other important things you did, but now you have a very important role and this job is just as important."

"What job?" she asked looking puzzled, "I don't do anything."

"Oh yes you do," I replied. "Without you, how can we teach our doctors and nurses about caring for somebody with your condition? That's your role, without you we wouldn't have a job either! You do know the expected outcome of your condition, don't you?"

She pondered this for a moment, "Maybe you're right," she said, "I hadn't thought of it that way. It will be sudden I do know, but time does drag so. I wish it was all over, I'm so tired and fed up with it all." At this juncture her priest arrived and I stood up to go.

"Thank you for your help," she smiled at me, I drew the curtains and left her to the padre.

As I walked away the ward staff nurse came up to me with a concerned look on her face.

"Can I ask what you were talking to Mrs Newbold about?" she asked politely.

"Dying," I replied. She made a face.

"Why?" she asked.

"Because that is what she wanted to talk about," I replied.

"She started on at me when I came on duty this morning and I told her not to be morbid," said the staff nurse.

"That's not being morbid," I said, "that's realistic. If she was eighteen it would be, but not at her age."

"Oh," she said, "you are clever. Have you studied psychology?"

"No, people," I replied. "Your subject!" She walked away smiling and nodding her head!

A week later Mrs Newbold collapsed and died without regaining consciousness as predicted. No, she had nobody else in her life who cared, and I could not be anything but glad for her.

I often found myself listening to the nursing staff who became distressed when confronted with problems and questions such as Mrs Newbold's dilemma. They couldn't answer them and were very embarrassed or dismissed the query as of little consequence, or they felt it was not their role to think about it. They would then, if they would take the trouble, refer this question to the padre, never wanting themselves to get caught up in another's emotions, but I felt, and often told nurses, that yes, this was part of the job, and they really did need to think about some of the more serious sides to life. Look into their own hearts and minds, be a lot more analytical, and try and understand what it would be like when they had to tread this path themselves on their own.

This episode made me realise that my place was in directly dealing with the sick. That's where I wanted to be to get fulfillment in my job, and not treating them by proxy which teaching the subject was! But being unable to see a way out of this, I then had to burn my boats and clear the decks as it were and point blank refused to do a two year university course offered to me by the director. Having had too much separation from my family when in the service I wanted no more of that way of life now, and had found considerable pleasure again in direct contact with sick people.

The director was quite indignant at my refusal and would offer me no other way out.

"You won't get any special treatment from me, even if you expect it," she said to me one day.

"Obviously," I replied, "I'll do my own thing even if it means leaving."

"Please yourself," she replied, and wiped her hands of me. She was pleasantly distant, and we conversed thereafter mainly in monosyllables.

So I went to work daily, got only some satisfaction out of it, wore out my new car a little more, and soldiered on. But I was determined to find an outlet for my frustrations. I think I must have been a pain in the neck to my colleagues even though most were on my side. Pam remarked after it all settled down that she got fed up with me, but we loved each other and our relationship was strong enough to take the strain. Then out of the blue came salvation.

Waking Up

I was going through the situations vacant page in the *Nursing Times* when I spotted a small ad for training nurses in acupuncture. "That's it," I shouted to Pam, "that's what I'll do, and go into private practice and treat people as I want to treat them."

I'd seen the results of the therapy when in the Far East and had been impressed, and immediately followed up the ad. It gave a telephone contact in Manchester, I phoned and spoke to a GP who was running the course, he asked a bit about me and said, "Yes you sound the right sort, send me £300" – a lot of money in 1970! – "and start in six week's time, eight weekend sessions and a certificate on completion, not the baffling Chinese sort," he said, "difficult for the average European to get his mind round that stuff, but a simple easy version!"

"Hang on," I replied, "I'm in education, what's your syllabus and other details?"

"I'll send them," he replied and a fortnight later received a scrap of A4 with a couple of sentences on it and that was that. And it was based on a medical model – not what I had expected. I'd been through a pill for every ill and wanted no more of it. I wanted to treat people, not their diseases.

Pam looked at it this scrap of A4 and said sarcastically, "Acupuncture has been around for thousands of years, you're not going to learn it in eight weekends," and I was forced to agree with her wisdom.

So my enthusiasm waned for a time, but a few weeks later, we were on holiday on the east coast and I was browsing through books in a good quality book shop and I found a book purely by chance on alternative medicine, took it down off the shelf and it actually fell open at traditional Chinese medicine! I started to read and found myself fascinated at the concepts therein regarding health and sickness. I knew straight away that some of the extraordinary concepts made a lot of sense to me. We were so busy in general medicine looking at disease, we failed to see how it had arisen in the first place and treated it, instead of the person with the disease. We failed so many times on both counts and the many treatments on offer often did harm, but the fact that we were doing something seemed to me was the main thing that mattered. I'd always wondered what one said to the patient after all the tests proved negative and the patient was told, 'So, you've got nothing wrong with you,' but the patient then says, 'Why don't I feel well then?'

There were going to be some answers then to these problems, I could feel in my bones!

On return from holiday I discussed my dilemma with my colleague Sophie. She had an open mind and knew what I had been going through, and at all times had been very supportive. Her main role in the department was tutor in charge of the post-registration training and she had very kindly co-opted me into some of her schemes, for which I was most grateful.

She said that she was always wary of the obviously opportunistic way fringe groups had of climbing on to bandwagons, and advised me to proceed with great caution and take qualified advice. But at all times she was encouraging, knowing my situation.

Sophie was Dutch; she had in her youth suffered under Nazi oppression in Amsterdam during the war, and so knew a bit about life. In one of her roles, she took a lot of interest in her expatriate community in this country, not only for social reasons, but also for helping with welfare problems.

One day she had to escort a young disabled Dutch man on a visit to an alternative medical clinic in London, and on her return told me that a lot of the other patients were waiting to see this doctor. The patients looked a little lost and abandoned – an odd lot, she observed – "Maybe that's the sort of patient you'll be dealing with if you go ahead, so be warned." However, to me, this was not discouraging at all; it was a helpful remark, but she qualified her statement by saying that she was sure I had the right skills to do this type of work.

So Sophie was a general adviser, comforter and encourager, both responses I needed at that time. Sophie was a very nice, comfortable person to be with, and I realise my good fortune in having had such a friend. She's dead now, but is one of those special people who lives in one's memory for being a wonderful human being.

She had awakened my interest again in acupuncture and I needed to get information about a proper course in Chinese medicine. I wrote to the *Daily Telegraph* who were at that time running a project in which they would answer employment questions. I requested them to research the subject, and a few days later received details of the British College of Acupuncture in London.

I wrote to them giving all my details and C.V. and after the usual acceptance procedure was accepted onto a pre-course year, an ab initio course in general medicine for nurses and others in professions supplementary to medicine, to learn the art of diagnosis, and on completion of this, if I passed, would be accepted onto a two year part-time acupuncture course.

4

A STUDENT AGAIN

It was 4.00 a.m. on Saturday 19th September 1979. I tramped down to Ely station to catch the train to London, hoping to arrive at the university at 8.30 a.m. to commence my ab initio course.

It was a cold rainy morning, the train was late and when it arrived it was scruffy and dirty, and as I sat in my seat and watched the fenland drift slowly past the window, I began to wonder just what on Earth I was doing, and why I was doing it!

I had to change trains at Cambridge; there were engineering works on the line and everything was delayed. I really could have got onto the next eastbound train and gone home and back to bed. But I gritted my teeth and got onto the London express – so called – and found myself sitting opposite a big scruffy individual who was smoking some foul concoction. As he finished each fag he opened the window wide, letting in a blast of freezing air, and threw the dog end out. I realised afterwards he was probably smoking cannabis, and didn't want to be apprehended by the authorities.

I arrived at the university on time and went straight into the common room as instructed, where a horde of apparently very ordinary-looking people were drinking disgusting coffee from a battered machine. After a roll call we were allocated to our group and escorted to our classroom, where we waited until the person in charge of us arrived.

He turned out to be a very pleasant elderly man with grey hair, Dr Redhead, a retired GP he said, who was going to turn our rather disparate lot of seventy-five souls into competent diagnosticians.

We were indeed a motley crowd, all in some ways in professions complementary to medicine, most of us aged from about thirty to sixty-five. Some were absolute nut cases, but the majority of us were looking for a degree of enlightenment having lost a lot of faith in the modern medicine machine.

We spent the first few sessions introducing ourselves and explaining our reasons for being there. This took up most of the morning, and a lot of funny ideas were expressed regarding expectations of what individuals wanted from the course, and in what direction they thought health care should go in future, and their part in it. It was interesting to hear all these persons' ideas; not all were very sensible, but to the individual himself!

One was of the opinion that all should be dosed from birth with large doses of vitamin C, another thought that everyone should have their bowel action recorded daily by filling in a form to make it legal – who was supposed to see it was not revealed, she was rather vague about that – and so on ad infinitum.

One or two students could not see why they should be on this course at all, but it was mandatory if one wanted to join the acupuncture course, after all they'd been at it for years and knew it all. Sadly this brigade was soon disillusioned when they found they did not know it all, and soon deserted the course, losing a lot of money in the process.

So the good Dr Redhead had his work cut out to bring this lot to heel and to teach the art of diagnosis, what and when to look, touch, feel, smell, hear, listen and so on, and to use diagnostic equipment sensibly and safely, and learn to trust our hunches and feelings, but always to be acutely aware that we were accountable.

He was a good teacher, and liberally sprinkled his lectures with appropriate anecdotes which held our attention. I realised at once that this was going to be a most interesting time, and so it proved to be. Unfortunately at the next week he did not arrive, and we learned later that he had suffered a massive heart attack and had not survived. But a replacement was soon found in a Dr Richard James, a very approachable young man who settled in well and received our approval.

After a few weeks the numbers began to dwindle when students discovered the amount of work they had to get through. There was a huge amount to study at home and I quickly realised I'd have to plan this very carefully indeed, and so set myself the task of completing one-and-a-half hours of study daily, and I'm proud to say that I kept to this schedule to the bitter end, working on holidays and even Christmas day itself, but in the end it paid off.

I began to find the weekend journeys rather onerous and looked for an easier route, and subsequently found that if I went part of the way by car to Royston and then caught the Kings Cross train, not only was it quicker, but Kings Cross was within walking distance to the college instead of, as before, having to use the tube from Liverpool Street.

In fact the walk in the morning and evening up Euston Road was quite a pleasure after sitting in lectures all day, but I was appalled at the amount of rubbish on the London streets, and what overseas students must have thought seeing people sleeping rough I hate to think. Frequently in the earlier part of the day I was accosted by scruffy souls down on their luck, asking for a pound to get some breakfast, so they said.

But my mind was on other things, and I was getting great pleasure with working with so many like-minded people, so that the work required did not distress me. The work was at a far deeper level than I had experienced on my teachers' course, but because of this I was more fortunate than most of my fellow students in that I did understand the language.

The course then was giving me a greater insight into medicine than I already had, but it was expensive, and with the travelling costs it was difficult for some people, and so slowly the number of dropouts increased and at the end out of the academic year; of the seventy-five we started with, only seventeen remained – quite an attrition rate – a lesson to all to count the costs in terms of both finance and time. I had to admit I could not have done this had I been doing my previous job of being in charge of pupil nurse training. I had little time there to think of other things then, so my director had, although she thought differently, done me a favour! I also felt that I was extremely lucky that I could afford the costs of the course, which had proved too much for many.

By working in the geriatric department at the hospital I had access to current medicine, and as the consultant in charge was sympathetic to my position in which I had been placed, I had the opportunity to be able to talk to the medical staff, pick their brains and get their comments on the problems we were set by our lecturers, which was a great help to me.

At the college we spent a lot of time in practical work, with role play and other techniques, learning all the little tricks and pitfalls in diagnosis, and I felt I was becoming quite expert at the subject – or so I thought!

One morning, Pam asked me to go upstairs before I left for the hospital to see what was wrong with my seventeen-year-old daughter Gillian. She worked as a receptionist at a local medical practice in the town and had complained on and off of a low-grade abdominal pain for the previous six months. This had been investigated by her GP, but he could find no reason for it. However, she had fallen out with another doctor at the practice who she claimed was making her life miserable by always criticising her work performance. We assumed she was trying to avoid work, as that day she was to be working for him on her own.

I had a quick look at her tummy and asked a few relevant questions and took her temperature, which all proved to be normal. I told her in tones of some asperity, that if she didn't stop moaning, one day she'd end up on the operating table and somebody would open her up to see if there was anything wrong, and then she'd know what pain really was!

At 9.30 a.m. Pam phoned me to say that Gillian was going to theatre at 10.30 with a suspected perforated appendix!

Oh dear, such is life! As I recounted this sorry tale to my colleagues in the common room, one said, "Couldn't you even diagnose an appendix, some course you're on I must say."

This brought me up quite sharply. I had said that sort of thing myself before this, but if you diagnose something then you've got to do something about it, and then live with the consequences if you're wrong. But diagnostics are not as easy as that, and if you are dealing with a loved one, who takes the can back then? That's doubly difficult.

Gillian had her surgery, survived and bore me no ill will, and she recovered quickly. We were all a bit more sympathetic thereafter as were the staff at the medical centre. We all learned a lesson from that!

So I soldiered on with the course, which was getting more and more intensive, but still most enjoyable, as we dug deeper into general medicine, but we were down to a small number now and were getting almost individual tuition! Those who had left, apart from cost, had not done their homework before enrolling and found out what was to be required of them, and what was involved.

So the exam came, two three-hour in-depth papers and a frightening viva where you had to scour your brain for answers, but I passed and was found fit to go into the main course in Chinese medicine, and to become an independent practitioner taking responsibility for my own actions, when I hopefully passed it!

It had been a hard year, but nowhere near as hard as the next two years were to be, which almost brought me to the edge of failure. But after a relaxing holiday in Scotland, on return I was ready to face the unknown, even if somewhat apprehensive.

5

TRADITIONAL CHINESE MEDICINE

I entered the new course with a considerable amount of trepidation. Most of my fellow students were holders of degrees in medicine or dentistry, there was one chap who was a consultant neurologist at a teaching hospital, so I wondered if I could keep up with such classmates, but I soon found they were as flummoxed as I! The concepts in TCM were so different to western thought, and the language translated from the Chinese was sometimes almost impossible to comprehend when such terms as excess, heat and cold, and so on meant such a different concept when used to describe symptoms. I found however a mad logic in some of these concepts when you got your brain into the right gear, but it required a great leap of faith and imagination to take them on board; it was not only the language, but these ideas were from a different culture which had developed long before ours had in the west when we lived in mud huts! It was a bit like trying to get to grips with a medieval mindset of the courts of Edward the third.

The language used in the common expressions we use, such as referring to butterflies in the stomach for nervousness, was called the sensation of a little pig running amok in the bowel! Lots of pigs in China but not a lot of butterflies! So it was cultural rather than semantics! Again, the sensation of a young fox clawing its way out of the chest, that is a nasty dose of tracheitis, and you've got the idea!

So apart from these expressions and the observation of reactions to illness, concepts such as yin and yang, excess and deficient, hot and cold, all had different connotations to those I had been brought up with, but were the bedrock of this form of medicine. It had after all, lasted some 2500 years and was still going strong, so there must be something in it for us poor flummoxed students, even though it left some of us gasping and indeed sceptical at times, until we got the idea! But however all these ideas were going to be used in the treatment of disease and the prevention of sickness and maintenance of health was to say the least, at that point, a total mystery!

Our lecturers, except for one or two, were very experienced people, but some of them, like so many experts in their own field, were not very good at getting the message across, and as a qualified teacher I sometimes sat with gritted teeth at the elementary mistakes in teaching that some made. I recall one episode before a weekly test, asking the lecturer what he was testing – was it the knowledge of facts and concepts, or the application of both or either of them? I remember him looking at me with a bemused expression on his face; one could almost hear his thought, 'So we've got a smart arse here have we!'

Fortunately we students, being by and large mature people, were able to help each other along, and we did have a lot of fun at times as we got to know each other better. Some real characters were beginning to emerge and some of those with some previous knowledge of the subject were able to unravel some of the concepts to we thicker ones in our motley crew. There was one chap who was blind, who was brilliant at explaining ideas to us where the lecturer had failed miserably; he'd been to China and had experienced the therapy at close quarters, and had a working knowledge of Mandarin as well.

The dean of the college, one Dr Royston Low, was pretty fluent in Chinese – or so he said – and would waffle on about some obscure concept for hours if you let him. He was a prolific writer; I have a number of his tomes with me as I write this, most are very helpful but to me still some are indecipherable. I have one, which he signed for me, and it caused a lot of roughish humour at the time.

I was working in the college clinic one day when the director, who happened to be the dean's wife, asked me if I had seen his latest book, looking at the book on offer I realised it was going to be a great help to me and said so. "You buy this then," she said, "and I'll get another one." The next week I saw the dean and asked him to sign my copy, which he did with a flourish. The next day in class I was the only one with a copy until he arrived with a pile of them under his arm.

"Did anyone want one?" he asked, whereupon naturally everybody did and purchased them forthwith.

Traditional Chinese Medicine

I suggested to them that they got the dean to sign their copies. "Might be worth a fortune one day," I said!

Sitting at the front of the lecture theatre was a great friend of mine; she was a night sister at one of the most famous of northern hospitals. She had bought one of the dean's books and had him sign it for her.

"Did he sign yours?" she asked me.

"Oh yes Marie," I replied, "he wrote something most complimentary in mine."

"What do you mean?" she asked.

"No, let me see what he has written in yours," I smirked, she showed me and I laughed. "Oh, is that all?" I said. "Well I'm sorry to say, if that's all he thinks of you, I'd give up now and go home."

"What do you mean?" she shrieked.

"Marie, the pen is mightier than the sword you know, what people think of you shows in what they write and what they feel about you! Words spoken mean little, they are just wasted on the desert air, but what is written is there for all to see," I said ponderously with a very straight face.

There was a frantic rush to get hold of my book to see what he'd written, but I wouldn't let it go, referring to inferior classmates and so on. After half an hour of bickering I relented. So, eyeing me suspiciously, she said, "Come on then, what did he write in yours?"

"Well as you know it's the impression one creates, isn't it, he wrote in your books 'With best wishes', I believe," I laughed.

"Yes," she spat back, "and what did he put in yours if I may ask?"

"Well if you must know, he wrote, and here I quote, 'With very best wishes', so there you are, that says it all doesn't it."

By this time all the others were falling about laughing. The bruise on my head did eventually fade!

We slowly built up a body of knowledge in the first year; the exams at the end were mainly about facts, not their application, and to my surprise I passed with a credit. I was now ready to go into my final year, but nemesis was waiting just around the corner.

Pam had been off sick from the hospital where she worked as a ward sister in the geriatric department. She had a neck problem; dealing with elderly patients over the years had taken its toll, and with all kinds of therapy little had been achieved. On one of her visits one evening to her GP she came out of the surgery looking a little puzzled and despondent.

"What's up?" I asked.

"I think he's trying to tell me I should give up work," she said tearfully.

"What do you think about that then?" I asked, knowing how much she loved her job.

"I'm fed up with the pain," she said. "I just don't know what to do."

"I'll go and ask him," I said and went back to talk to him.

"Were you saying to my wife that it's time to give up work?" I asked him.

"What do you think?" he replied.

"Oh no, that's your decision, not mine. She's got to have somebody to blame and it's not going to be me."

He made a face, but he was a compassionate man. "Yes," he said, "I do think it's time. She won't be any easier until she stops work, it's just too heavy a job."

"Will you tell her?" I asked. "If so I'll go and get her." And so he did tell her, hesitantly but kindly; she was one of his better ward sisters at the hospital where he was a non-resident physician, and he knew her capabilities and the standard of her work, and said he was sorry to see her go.

After we left, she was rather shocked and said something uncomplimentary about him. I didn't correct her; that would have been me I thought, had it been my decision.

So she left the hospital to a pension, but our income was now halved and I needed to think seriously about the future and if I could afford to carry on with the course. But fortunately my bank manager was understanding and loaned me the money to carry on, "If you are going to pass!" he said. "Will you pass?" he asked.

I laughed, "With that sort of debt I've got no option, have I!" I replied.

By the time I had got through the next term I felt I was getting to grips with the concepts, but there was a nagging doubt in my mind about the true efficacy of the therapy. I still had nagging doubts in my mind about its ability to change one's life around when afflicted with ill health.

A lot of others in the class were of the same opinion and wanted to see evidence of success. They wanted to see some dramatic incident of the sort we saw when the steroids first were used, and arthritic patients could walk again (what they didn't want to see, however, were the disastrous side effects of the drug that came later!). But we were doing our 200 hours stint in the college clinic and now hoped to see evidence – we'd heard all about it, now let's see it for ourselves! And out of the blue for me came the irrefutable proof.

One day when out with the caravan, I hurt my back trying to move the beast out of a rut and strained my sacro-iliac joints, which gave me a lot of back pain, on top of the chronic low-grade back pain that almost all nurses complained of due to lifting heavy patients. In those days patient hoists were few and far between.

One morning I arrived at the clinic wondering if I could get through the day because of the pain, and after a couple of hours I'd had enough and went to sit and rest in the office. The clinic director came looking for me.

"What are you doing? We've got a lot of patients to see," she said. I got up to follow and she realised that I had a problem, "You've hurt your back, haven't you?" she said. "Come on, hop onto a couch and we will have a look at you."

"Who's we?" I asked timidly.

"The students of course," she replied testily, "come on."

"I don't want to be seen by someone like me," I replied.

"Get on the couch," she commanded. So, discretion being the better part of valour, I did as I was told.

The students and their tutor examined and prodded, asked all the right questions and then stuck a lot of needles in my back.

They were not very skilful, the doctors on the course seemed to the most ham fisted, but after half an hour they walked off leaving me to my own devices. After a few minutes of this enforced solitude I'd had enough, got up and pulled my clothes on and went and sat down back in the office and promptly went to sleep!

The director came back, woke me up, checked I was alright, and then directed me to a couple of new patients to be clerked.

The afternoon had gone quickly, and at four o'clock I had to leave to get to Kings Cross to get my train. I left in a hurry, rushed to the overcrowded tube at Hyde Park Corner, and eventually got to the station just in time to catch my train, sat down in the nearest seat, and suddenly realised that for the first time in weeks I had no backache! So it did work – so much for scepticism!

Suddenly, academically I was beginning to find it difficult. I was on a plateau and couldn't find my way off it. Somehow I'd got stuck; I knew all the words by now, but could not think quickly enough to put them into action. This block lasted until the spring term, and I began to feel that by no stretch of the imagination was I going to be ready for the finals in June.

The work had piled up and I was spending hours trying to study with little improvement. Maybe I was trying too hard, but in the end thought I would have to withdraw from the course. Pam told me to pack it in; she was getting fed up with my complaining, and I was sorely tempted to do that. However, again help was at hand and from a most unexpected source!

One morning as I went to work, 'Thought for the Day' was on Radio Four. I regularly listened to this daily, it was usually some anodyne waffle, but this day it was the Bishop of Peterborough, Bill Westwood, giving the talk. He was usually the best speaker who did this slot, and usually I rather liked his talks as he always had something to say that was interesting and to-the-point.

He told the story of a family member of his who had reached an impasse in her life. He briefly described her predicament which, was threatening her whole future. Somewhere he knew he had an article in a book which he felt would answer her problem, and he went up in the loft to find it. Whilst he was looking, he came across a sermon he'd written as a theological student years ago in response to his director of studies, who'd threatened him with dismissal from his college if he didn't get away from the sports field and do the set work, and he was weeks behind, so his director said that if he did a really good sermon he could stay, otherwise he was out.

This sermon was based on the New Testament account of the risen Christ standing on the shore of Lake Galilee and telling the disciples who had caught no fish all night to cast out their nets into the deep and they would find plenty of fish. That's what they did, and it is said, so many fish were caught that their nets broke.

That, declared the good bishop, was what his relative needed – have a go or you'll never know!

This story hit me right between the eyes, this was what I needed, have a go or the whole of the previous three years would have been wasted. At that point I relaxed for the first time in months, I had my answer!

When I got to the hospital, one of my colleagues said to me, "What's the matter with you? You look very cheerful." I told her what had happened, she said, "Thank goodness, we all thought you were going to pack it in, well done."

So in June I took the exams, and very gruelling they were too, and hoped to pass. I never told the bishop. When I next saw him at the nurses' prize giving, he was surrounded by the upper ranks of the NHS and I couldn't get near him, but I'm sure he would have been pleased that one lost soul who'd lost his bottle benefited from his two-minute talk. The bishop is dead now, but I will always think of him with gratitude for his thoughts that spring morning.

6

INTERLUDE

So I soldiered on in the geriatric department awaiting my exam results. Things were changing in the nursing profession. I was not keen on what I saw was happening. It seemed to me that we were concentrating on improving the lot of the staff and the patient was coming second. Yes there was a lot that could be done for both, but there was a lot of talk, but little action. We needed to be dragged into the twenty-first century, but how this was to be done I had only a hazy idea. One senior member of the Royal College of Nursing wrote a book describing the all graduate profession he would like to see; the then-Minister of Health, who was ill in hospital at the time, was given this as bedtime reading, swallowed it whole and off we went, and a whole new system was developed without the state-enrolled nurse and a huge lot of other changes as well, and everybody apart from those it would affect most climbed onto the bandwagon. The future of the profession was laid out in tablets of stone, and somehow we non-businesspeople had to deal with this very expensive and time-consuming exercise – the problem being running the profession as a business, which it certainly was not.

We were not unused to dealing with graduates from other disciplines, often those who were disillusioned with what they were doing in their chosen sphere, and wanting a more caring role in life. These people were a joy to deal with; they had a different attitude to life, having seen a chunk of it, and also had a touch of scepticism which enabled us as teaching staff to often enjoy great moments of debate with many of these clever people, rather than the wide eyed acceptance of some of the things teenagers saw who were without the knowledge or ability to question. Would this attitude be transferred to nurses, we wondered?

But the eventual demise of the SEN struck a severe blow to the nursing workforce, until it did eventually recover somewhat and upgraded them to SRN after a compressed course if they were suitable.

Interlude

Whilst I was awaiting my exam results, an ex-colleague of mine from the RAF was appointed to the staff as tutor. He lived a few miles away from me and we started to share the journey to work each day, which was financially beneficial to us both. John was a nice man, unmarried, a reader in the Church of England and churchwarden at his local parish church, so we had a lot in common. As a single man he had many interests, including glider flying, stamp collecting, railways and so on, and could talk quite authoritatively about most of these activities.

He was, however, a bit of a mad cap in a car, and when driving with him I was always glad, and sometimes not a little surprised, when we reached our intended destination in one piece! He was slightly lax in his observation of the speed limits, and seemed to be quite surprised when I asked him to slow down, and wondered what all the fuss was about! He appeared to be oblivious of his passenger when driving – they were there only to be talked at – and his car, not well-maintained, was noisy, and to cover up the noise he had his radio on full blast to drown the mechanical noise. Also, his heater was permanently jammed in the full on position, so summer and winter alike he drove with the window wide open, which of course added to the noise. Although he had an interest in everything, he had little interest in his own health, and sadly ill health caught up with him in the end and he had a most unpleasant terminal illness.

He caused a lot of amusement in the common room, however, and was well loved as a member of the staff. The students thought he was the bee's knees, and wouldn't hear a word against him. His enthusiasm for trivia had no bounds, but was sometimes misplaced. I recall that one day we were driving at speed along one of the elevated roads in the fens along the main drainage river near his home. It was a narrow road; I rarely drove at more than 40 mph on this stretch, this being a most unwise activity in that one mistake when dodging the many sugar beets that had fallen off farmers' lorries onto the carriage way, which was a well known hazard in those parts, it was possible for one to end up in the river! And one day, fortunately I was not with him, he did skid, plunged into the river at speed, and in trying to extricate himself through the broken windscreen, swam in a disorientated state to the opposite bank, climbed out very wet and cold, and had to walk some half a mile to the nearest bridge along the opposite bank to get help. The emergency services, however, were alerted by a passing motorist – they got there quickly, and found the car twenty foot down, managed to get it out in a hurry to find nobody in it, and started scouring the river for two people, because somebody told them that usually two persons were in the car when they saw it in the mornings! He had been marking exam papers the night before and had them with him; all of these were recovered from the wreck eventually, ruined of course, and the poor students had to take the exam again, much to their chagrin, but forgave poor John as was expected. I think the exam must have been doctored in the circumstances, as they all passed, but John lost his car and replaced it with an even more disreputable heap!

John one morning was doing his usual seventy-five; I was clinging on for dear life, when suddenly he shouted above the roar of the engine, "Get your wing up."

I nearly jumped out of my skin! I shouted back, "What the blazes are you on about?"

"That idiot in the crop-spraying kite over there is inept. He's going to crash in a minute, shouldn't be allowed to fly!" I looked to where he was pointing, hand off the wheel; the crop sprayer in question looked very competent to me flying along the rows of crops, turning steeply at the end of each, but compared to John's expertise who was I to give an opinion?

As we came home that evening still hurtling along in the heat, the radio local news was being broadcast, at full volume of course. There was a news flash to say that a crop spraying aircraft that morning had crashed near where we were, and the pilot had been killed. Well, you'd have thought John had won the pools; a great shout of "Told you so!" accompanied by a delighted grin. He dined out on that for weeks! He was not a vindictive man, just a bit thoughtless and daft at times! But he was also a self-declared expert on electronics and all the latest gadgets, such things as video players and cine cameras and so on. They were no mystery to John!

He started to encourage colleagues to make films and recordings for teaching aids to start with; they were dreadful, but he was proud of them, and he improved a bit as he went along. But nothing really worthwhile was produced; he had so many fingers in so many pies that it was very difficult to get John together with all the equipment needed at the same time. At that time we had a brand new geriatric department built. The old one stood empty with all its equipment for some time before it was demolished, and John thought this would make a good set to produce very simple films for the training of auxiliary staff to emphasise simple but important points in the care of elderly patients.

One thing he and a colleague wanted to get over was the importance of maintaining dignity and privacy for the sick when performing their natural functions. He asked me if I would play the part of an elderly patient – I didn't look old then, thirty years ago! I was to be dressed in pyjamas, dressing gown and slippers, trundled from the ward on a portable commode to the toilet, and left to get on with it. This was to emphasise the correct way to transport patients safely, and when I was ready, the accompanying nurse would ask if I was ready, then open the door, collect my toilet things and towel, pull the flush and so back to bed with a satisfied, relieved patient. Well that was the plan!

John of course was in total control, giving a running list of instructions; he was camera man, editor, continuity man, voice over and so on.

They eventually got me to the toilet after a number of retakes; I'd done the necessary and was now ready. On cue I called, "Ready nurse." And in came the nurse, picked up my bits and pieces making sure nothing was left behind, and went to pull the chain.

What we had forgotten was that the water was turned off and some of the plumbing removed. As the poor nurse pulled the chain there was an almighty crash, and part of the cistern came crashing down with a great shower of rust all over us. The nurse collapsed on the floor, shrieking with laughter, shouting, "They've turned the bloody water off!" John however courageously continued filming, we went back to the department, looked at the film and fell about laughing. We did use the film, but to show what you should not do!

John was a great friend to have and always good for a laugh when things went pear-shaped. As an unmarried man he was often off-putting to women, he certainly did not understand them. I felt he was a bit frightened of the ladies. He was well known in the health authority for some of his more outlandish ideas and his injudicious comments, but I'm sure he had no enemies, and we indulged his mad ways and missed him when he left us.

Even on his retirement party he dropped another clanger, in his farewell speech. With a captive audience, he lambasted us all for not visiting him in one of his admissions to another hospital. Then as I pointed out to him after the party was over, "But you never told us you were going to be admitted, we thought you were off on one of your schemes."

He was quite unabashed, "Oh, didn't I," he said, "must have forgotten!"

None of us would ever forget JGH as we knew him, one of life's great characters.

By the end of August my finals results were due, and after a nail-biting week they arrived: a plain brown envelope from the dean congratulating me on passing the exam and giving details of how much to pay to be registered! So it was now time to seriously think of how to cope with the future. I now had two good qualifications I could use for this, but the choice had to be considered with care; stay in nursing, or take a part-time post and practice acupuncture for the rest of the time.

I had certainly travelled hopefully and got to the end of my three years' journey, and now which path would I tread in future?

My life at the hospital had to continue, for the time being, not being a very fulfilling role; I felt that I was still nursing the sick by proxy, and had little if any authority – far less than I had as a tutor in charge of pupil nurse training.

I do not think the then-director realised just what she had done to my self-esteem. I was grateful to the reaction of my colleagues for their congratulations and best wishes – they'd taken an interest all through the three years as I told them about my studies – but the director had a closed mind and would not even discuss it with me. I still felt very resentful because of her action in depriving me of a role commensurate with my abilities.

However, again help was at hand. The director resigned, we were told for health reasons, and a search for a new director was begun. This went on for some four months and once again poor old Jack took over until a successful candidate was appointed, and to my delight he turned out to be my ex C.O. from the RAF, who I had worked with for over a year in the service and with whom I had had an excellent relationship. The future looked brighter now, and I could plan knowing that he would advise and help in any way possible. It was going to be for all that a long haul, but he helped me along the way, and for that I will always be grateful to him for his consideration.

7

BUILDING A PRACTICE

The new year began with a change of lifestyle for Pam and I. I had started to see one or two patients in our home town of Ely, in a small rented consulting room over a health food shop in the town on Saturday mornings.

A senior RAF officer in the medical branch, who had taken the same acupuncture course as myself some years previously, had a small private practice in the town. She was posted overseas and asked me if I would take over her few patients when she went.

I had known her first when she did a locum at the sick quarters in RAF Tobruk in Libya, and we had got on well from the start. It was with some surprise to me that she asked a newly-qualified person with limited alternative experience to take her patients, but I was most grateful for this as it gave me a real jump start. Unfortunately, the town was not ready for me, and even with this help it was very slow going! It was rather disappointing, but thirty years ago acupuncture was a relatively new import to this country. We are a very conservative race; many classified the therapy as, if not unbelievable, making little sense, some sections of the nonconformist church and fundamentalists called it devil-inspired, and I fell out with a good friend of mine of many years who thought I'd allied myself to the devil. Sadly he never spoke to me again!

Initially I had one quite dramatic success. My daughter, who by now was married to an RAF serviceman and living on a base in Norfolk, phoned me one day and asked me if I would treat her knee. She'd had trouble with her knee for some years, and when she worked at the health centre had had it investigated by an orthopaedic consultant and one or two other experts, none of whom could pinpoint the problem, even with scans and so on. Their only suggestion to her was to have the kneecap removed – a patelectomy. At the time I thought this was a bit drastic and asked her if she had seen patients who had had the operation done. She said she had, so I asked her if these patients were any better for the surgery, she said that they were not. "So there's your answer," I said. So now it was up to me to work the miracle!

Reluctantly I agreed to treat her when next she visited us. I am always aware of the hazards of treating ones nearest and dearest; it often goes pear-shaped and you haven't then got a leg to stand on. In her case I prayed that she would have a leg to stand on after the session! She arrived. I looked at and felt her knee and found the painful bit, and inserted two needles at the prescribed points for knee pain. Suddenly she said she felt a sensation of a mouse running up the back of her leg, and then the pain went, never to appear again. That was thirty-five years ago, and she has since had no more trouble with that knee.

This episode really cheered me up, but recognising that it takes more than one swallow to make a summer. I had to restrain myself and not become over-confident, and indeed over the years I've had great success at times with the previously untreatable patient with conventional medicine, and also howling failures.

Seeing patients now was different. It seemed strange taking money from people for treatment; I'd been handing out treatment for nothing, paid for by the state of course, for years. I was embarrassed at first and often forgot to ask them for my fee, and I had to pluck up courage sometimes to remind them of the fee I expected. As the practice didn't grow, my bank manager who had been a great help said to me one day, "You need to find somewhere with more chimney pots. Working one day a week in a small town is not going to get you anywhere, professionally or financially. It is time to move on."

The Peterborough Development Corporation at that time was encouraging businesses to locate to the city and ran an organisation called the Enterprise Scheme to give help and advice to those who thought they could start up on their own. I thought this might be of value, so made an appointment to see one of their consultants. These people were either senior members of big commercial banks, or those in financial institutions who had knowledge of new business, and I spent a most informative afternoon with a consultant from one of the major UK city banks. He listened carefully, asked a lot of questions, and in conclusion advised me to go ahead with my plans. He said I couldn't lose, so long as I followed advice both financially and professionally, but I must get an accountant and plan for an eleven-month financial year.

"Why eleven months?" I asked him.

He replied, "You'll be on your own, it gets very lonely and working with sick people is a strain," as I well knew, but I needed at least a month's holiday a year, as he put, to stave off madness!

He gave me advice on property rent or purchase, and also on tax affairs, and I ended up with four sheets of A4, which he said was for my bank manager, to see that I'd done my homework if I wanted to borrow money and open a business account. I had not realised how much there was to do, but this meeting cleared up a lot of unanswered questions and certainly eased my way into business. As he pointed out, "It's all about making a living, but you've got the right attitude by seeking advice and the right professional qualifications to succeed."

The next step was to rent premises that were acceptable, but when I got home that evening, to my amazement, Pam announced that she'd put our house on the market. I knew what our house in Ely meant to her; it was our first property and we'd had it modified as it was being built to our own specifications and made a very comfortable home of which we were both proud. I was very moved by this, but as she said, we were not going to make a proper living in a small town like Ely in those days. So we started looking for property to buy. I didn't want to rent; commercial rents were quite expensive, and that would take a large chunk of income as well as the mortgage we were paying.

It proved very difficult at first. The estate agents were helpful, but there was not a lot of suitable property available. After a week or two of fruitless searching, I then thought I should question the right of a house owner to get planning permission if we did find a property and have it modified. The council were helpful with this but somehow it seemed too easy! After one of our fruitless visits to the city to see a property recommended to us by the estate agents, when we got home there was an answer phone message – would we phone the agents? They had a client with cash at the office, who wanted a house urgently. He was a solicitor and was moving to the town in the near future. We invited them to come round at once, they fell for the house immediately, just what they wanted, it was November now, could we be out by Christmas? I looked at Pam and said, "I'll get a hospital house pro temp," she nodded, and we agreed, and the deal was done.

Next day I went to see the accommodation officer at the hospital to ask if we could rent a hospital house. He said those houses were only for people to whom they were offering posts, "so no, sorry, you'll have to rent somewhere else."

I went back to my office in the school of nursing and collapsed in a heap. Now what? I then had a sudden thought – the planning people had been too dismissive of my worries about information about modifying property when I spoke to them before. I spoke to another chap on the phone this time, he told me that their previous information was right, and if I was worried about it, an osteopath who had a practice just over the road from the hospital had built his own practice, why not go and talk to him. I was desperate, so went straight over to his property to find a 'for sale' sign on it – the owner was retiring and wanted to downsize. A fully-equipped set of rooms including toilet, waiting room, consulting room and so, and he was asking the same price that we were selling our house for!

I phoned Pam, she came straight up on the next train, and we did the deal there and then. We were in business. And so, everything seemed to be coming together at last!

We had planned to spend the Christmas holiday at a hotel in Bournemouth owned by my eldest son's father-in-law and his two business partners. Our proposed move threw things into a bit of a muddle, but we decided to go ahead and it was eventually arranged that we would move to Peterborough into the practice on January 3rd 1983.

The holiday was a bit of a disaster, we were on edge because of the imminent move, but both my son and daughter-in-law did their best to entertain us and took us out to see the sights. The other guests at this small hotel were a bit pathetic. One woman spent the whole holiday moaning to anybody who would listen about her toothache, and spent the time eating Panadol tablets washed down with copious glasses of gin, and a party of elderly men, all single and of doubtful sexual orientation, spent the whole time tanking up on Red Barrel. After Boxing Day lunch, when we were all in the bar having a post-prandial drink with mine host, one of these men vomited his whole stomach contents over all the guests, then indulged in a long complaint with the others of the iniquity of the brewery in providing a bad barrel of beer! It didn't occur to these idiots that as none of the rest of us drinking the same beer were affected, and that their problem could possibly be caused by their over indulgence. They had been drinking solidly since they'd arrived at the hotel after all!

So we were glad when the holiday was over, and headed home ready for the fray.

It was a sad day leaving our home in Ely. This was the first house we had bought and had it modified to our own specification, and now we were moving into a second-hand property which, although the same age as our Ely house, had no modifications in it to bring it up to date. It needed a proper kitchen and bathroom, but we had made the decision to go into business and the goodies would have to wait.

The 'new' house, having been owned by an elderly couple now in poor health, was carpeted in the most outlandish-coloured excellent quality carpet, yellow with red and blue roses. In an open-plan house it looked like an enormous flowerbed, but it was too good to throw out and we had to wait some six years before we had the money to replace this dreadful thing. The wallpaper was little better; that went at the same time as the carpet, but we learned to live with it!

The garden was extensive and had been neglected for a good two years, and I had to spend hours burning the thick layer of leaves from next door's overhanging plane tree. I eventually took six large dustbin bags of ash down to the town dump.

The office and its rooms were ideal, but again with appalling canary yellow walls and a green carpet. Everyone who came into it looked as if they had a bad case of jaundice, but this was easily remedied with a few tins of paint and a new carpet to my choice of colour. When it was finished it looked very smart indeed, and worth all the hard work.

I bought new furniture for the room, and with the help of a colleague we arranged it all ready for the business I planned to start within the month. However, poor Pam had to sort out the house, which was in need of a lot of love to turn it into the comfortable home we ended up with as the years rolled by.

So I put a small advert in the local evening paper, and almost at once the enquiries began to come in. I had set my working week for all day Saturday and each evening six to nine, apart from Sunday. Pam was concerned that I would not be able to keep this up for long because of my increasing workload at the hospital, and indeed it was tiring. With a new director at the school, he was finding me a lot of interesting things to do, for which I was grateful, but I was finding I had less and less spare time.

Initially most of the patients who attended my new practice had experienced ill health for years, all other treatments had failed and they wanted a miracle. I was honest with them, and always told them although I could help them to possibly experience their problem in a different way, a cure would not be possible. The therapy was not about cure, but among other things changing lifestyle, avoiding aggravating factors, and modifying their reaction to their complaint. But most had read in those early days, and seen on television, and read in *The Sun* of miraculous interventions in people's lives by acupuncture, most of it being fantasy.

I remember well one of my first patients; he was a most uncouth man and was quite rude to me when he phoned to make an appointment. "I've got a bad hip," he shouted, "everybody who has had a go at it has done me no good, I don't suppose you will do any better but I'll come and see if you're as bad as the rest!" *Thanks very much*, I thought. But I agreed to see him; he was quite right, I couldn't do anything, he needed a hip replacement and I told him so.

"Thought so," he crowed, "you are as bad as the rest, all they want to do is to cut you up," and with that he threw his fee at me and stormed out! I never saw him again. At this stage of my career I was not experienced enough to realise just what was possible with the therapy, but sensible enough to know that, 'to cure sometimes, to relieve often, but to comfort always' was the most important thing. At least, that was my ambition!

After two years of full-time working at the hospital and the time I was giving to the practice, I was really beginning to feel the strain, so I asked Roy the director if I could start to use my leave entitlement so as to ease the strain. This gave me now four days hospital and two plus in the practice, which was a considerable improvement. Roy was being very helpful, and we negotiated a working pattern that not only benefited me, but also the school of nursing. In fact Roy was becoming an excellent director, and was able to negotiate in the corridors of power the many changes that lay ahead for the profession with some clout.

As my practice grew, I was also being more involved with professional duties at the hospital. I became the press spokesman for our branch of the Royal College of Nursing, and one or two other jobs came my way, one such being giving recruiting talks at local schools. None of these jobs were particularly onerous, but all helped to repair my shattered self-esteem, which had been so badly bruised by the previous director. At that time in 1979 we were trying to get a better salary, and as negotiations with government appeared to have stalled, I decided as the press person of the RCN to do a mass postal lobby of our local M.P.

This proved to be so successful that he came down to address the membership in the recreation centre, all 250 nurses at the hospital were present and proceeded to give him a hard time! Each response to a question of course got a politician's answer, which was only words. After a time he got a bit fed up, and asked what really was the problem, because it was obvious that his audience felt his answers had little credibility. "Is it staff shortage?" he asked wearily. A roar of assent greeted this, the headquarter based RCN rep turned to me and asked if we were short of staff, I replied that we were actually over the top by twenty nurses. I received a roar of disapproval, but then explained it wasn't total numbers that was the problem, but establishment.

We now had extra leave, more courses which were mandatory, a shorter working week, the pattern of care was changing, a shorter bed occupancy and more acutely ill patients who were often sent home prematurely, and then had to be readmitted etc. At the start of the NHS, the establishment was one nurse to one-and-a-half beds, but it was now five beds with the one nurse. This statement was greeted by the members with approval, not that I think they understood, but somehow trusted me to get it right! The M.P. said he had not realised that, so he'd look into it with the minister. So the meeting was successful and we felt we had achieved something.

But then a few days later, the local press phoned me about the pay negotiations. "Have you seen the national papers today?" the reporter asked.

"Yes I have, so what?" I replied,

"Did you see that the bishops of the C of E have received a pay rise of

18.5% and all you are asking for is 4%? Do you not think that saving lives is more important than saving souls?"

I thought for a moment, how do you respond to an argument put forward by a grown man with all the intelligence and acumen of a ten-year-old? "Do you know how many bishops there are?" I asked.

"I really don't," he replied warily.

"Well, there are about one hundred in all," I replied and went on, "Do you know their salary?" I asked him.

"Well no," he said.

"It's about £6000 plus expenses," I replied. I knew this because a friend of mine was a clergyman and we had discussed this previously.

"Oh," he said, but I'd not finished with this idiot yet!

"Do you know how many nurses there are?" Again, he did not. "A quarter of a million, so you think about that," I told him, and I put the phone down. However he got his quote in the paper that evening – he got some idiot to agree with his ridiculous question. '"More important to save lives that souls" says local ambulance chief!' said the headline. I'm glad it wasn't me he quoted!

I was beginning to enjoy life at the hospital now that we were under a more trusting and benevolent directorship, and was given more and more responsibilities, things that my colleagues were unsure about and didn't want to be involved in. My next role was to be appointed as a safety representative under the Health and Safety at Work Act. I'd always been interested in legal matters and had to attend various courses to get familiar with the Act's workings. The concept of HASAWA was first-class, I felt, and would go a long way to solving some of the problems in industry, even if it did not always appear relevant to hospital ward work. But, of course, unless it was applied in the spirit of the legislation, instead of the way it has been highjacked at times, and used by the ignorant and devious as a means of avoiding responsibilities, and those who used it for personal reasons and used it to be lazy and to avoid doing what they didn't want to do, it could only be a good thing to regulate the work place.

One of my first experiences of the Act occurred when a colleague went to the butchers and came back with six sheep hearts to dissect in the classroom. I heard about this and pointed out that there were now a lot of regulations governing use of animal tissue, and although this was not covered specifically by the Act, the Act was quite clear about the use of correct facilities. Other legislation was involved in this, giving details of the places in which this could be done, disposal of waste, cleaning agents to be used, wipe-down surfaces, adequate protective clothing and so on. A great squark of protests greeted my comments followed by the well-used phrase, 'This is what we've always done'.

"Well, not anymore," I replied. "Take it to the lab. I'm not trying to stop you, just do it in the right risk-free place." There was a particular report that had been issued on the subject of dealing with dead tissues which was used by the laboratory, so I duly went to talk to the senior technician of the lab and request information. He was not only unwilling to talk to me about it, but reported the school to the management claiming that we were cutting up dead tissue in the school without the correct facilities. So much for cooperation among departments in the NHS. I found this attitude extensive in the NHS, and it would appear to be common to this day!

It's interesting to think how things had turned out for me; had I not been eased out of my career earlier, I would not have been doing those things now which stretched me intellectually, indeed a lot further than teaching pupil nurses. But with HASAWA, employment law, common law and so on, I found it necessary to look at all these things now when advising on the day to day running of the department and its affairs. I spent a lot of time poring over textbooks on these subjects until I was certain I knew what I was talking about.

My next course was to Dudley Polytechnic as part of my five-year nurse teachers' refresher. This course was on the production of visual aids for use in the classroom. I produced at this excellent establishment a tape slide programme on accident prevention, and was most flattered when the polytechnic kept a copy for their own use as an example of how it should be done. Needless to say, this was of course with the expert help of one of the tutors; he'd been a photographic interpretation officer in the RAF, so what he didn't know about the subject you could have put on a sixpence!

The course at Dudley had for me an unexpected and bizarre incident, which left me aware that places and buildings can absorb emotions and feelings of the people who in the past had inhabited them. There are places for example in the high peak district of Derbyshire, when the weather is dull windless and misty, you can almost see the prehistoric nature of the landscape and feel the effect it must have had on our ancestors, it's also an area where you can't trust your compass to give a reliable reading!

The Sunday afternoon before I started my course at the tech, Pam and I had taken the caravan with us, intending to stay on for a week after the course. We were out in the country and I saw a road sign to Hednesford. This was the RAF unit where I'd done my two months square bashing in 1954. I'd not realised that we were in that vicinity. Hednesford was on the top of a hill in Cannock Chase, a place of memories, bitter weather, crude screaming drill instructors, food fit for animals, and lots of misery!

So we set out to find it, and after a long haul found a road which I thought I recognised from all those years ago; the unit now long gone, but the area was being cleared of all the detritus of military occupation and was being turned into a country park.

We walked through the gate, the roads were still there. I was able to recognise the location of the various buildings. We walked up the long road to the top of the small hill in the middle of the area, and stood overlooking the place where the unit had been, now devoid of buildings. It was a windless, dull afternoon, very quiet, no birds, and it was summer, and I remembered, looking at this dismal scene, the misery I and a lot of others suffered as National Service men. Suddenly Pam grabbed my arm.

"What's that noise?" she said. I listened and heard it, the sound of marching men and shouted commands. Pam heard it too and recognised what it was. It was genuine! It took me right back all those years ago to the misery of National Service. The hair stood up on the back of my head, "Come on," I shouted, "let's get out of here, this is not nice." We drove away quickly, not a pleasant experience.

I attended other courses on drug and alcohol addiction, and attended one conference in London near Victoria station. The conference centre was not far from Westminster Catholic Cathedral. It was a lovely spring day with all the trees coming into leaf, and London was alive with tourists. In the lunch hour I wandered down the road to the cathedral, having never seen it before, except on television.

On the steps before the church were some winos, big rough men, decidedly scruffy and all drinking out of unlabelled bottles. Two policemen were keeping a careful eye on them, but I was rather annoyed that these people were here in front of all these foreign tourists, and wondered just what they must have thought of these four outside a place of worship. I turned my head away and did my best to ignore them, and out of curiosity went into the cathedral to see the sights. I didn't think much of the architecture, if you compared it with the abbey, but it was quiet and peaceful.

A mass was being said in one of the side chapels, I paused to listen as the celebrant began to read the parable of the Good Samaritan. He had a lovely, well-modulated Irish voice. It was quite entrancing to stand there and listen. Eventually I looked at my watch and realised I had only ten minutes left to get back to the conference centre.

I walked out into the warm sunshine, the crowds were still milling around. The winos were still there. I had to walk close to them to get by, one raised his bottle to me in drunken salute, and said something.

Suddenly I saw their problem; I was a little calmer now, my annoyance ameliorated by the voice of the priest. They've cracked it, I thought, their problems all solved in their bottles. What could I offer them better than the oblivion they found in their booze? Unemployment, mortgages, kids, commuting, and all the normal cares of life, they'd solved it for themselves in their own way – not a very pleasant way, but that was not my business.

As I walked away, I felt a little ashamed of my intolerance, and it troubled me for some time. Would He, in whose name that great cathedral had been built, would He have just walked away from those men? I doubt it.

Some days after this foray into the great metropolis and back at the hospital, I was asked to do a lesson on communications. When I asked what they meant by this, I received a rather wooly reply: "Well, you know, getting the message across!" Quite a subject to cram into one session!

I decided that would best be done by taking a party of these senior students to the ward and teaching them how to talk and listen to those patients who were willing to talk; not all are, and often what they don't say is as important as what they do say, and it was not common for nursing staff to be allowed to stand and chat, often considered to be a bit of a time-wasting exercise. I did not agree with this contention. We always seemed to me, and more so as I became more experienced, to be the result again of the pill for every ill syndrome; if you've cured the body, that's what they are in hospital for, and that is what we've done! So get on with your work!

I took these students to the medical ward to talk to a wild fowler who'd had a heart attack whilst working at night in the marshes on the washes. I warned them that if the conversation became too intrusive they must stop their inquisition at once and I would take over, but showing a surprising amount of sensitivity, and following the guidelines I'd set for them, they did very well, and the result of their conversation eventually contributed in great measure to the patient's complete recovery. The patient was a retired businessman, a widower, who had always loved the countryside and country pursuits, and on retirement after his wife died had bought a cottage by the marshes. He spent most of his time fishing or shooting, he told us, out with his dog. But one night out on the marsh, he'd suffered crushing chest pain, managed to get home and called the ambulance, and was admitted to the coronary care unit with a heart attack. He'd been treated well he said, and was now pain-free. However, what he did not tell us was that he was not now improving. The medical staff had told me prior to this exercise that they were concerned that he appeared to be on a plateau, and hopefully he was not going to regress or not make any further progress at all; if so he would become a chronic heart patient with little quality of life, supported by medication and with a very limited future as to what he could do. Certainly he would be unable to go wild fowling again.

I did not tell the students this, but let them ask about his life, which he was pleased to talk about. I prompted them quietly, 'Ask them about his dog'.

He had a black Labrador he said that he'd trained as a gun dog, and believe it or not, he called him Rover! His best friend, he said, and would say no more.

It was obvious that we'd got to the nub of the matter, I took one of the students aside, I knew she liked dogs, and told her to talk to him about her dog then see what happened. She talked for a while about her dog, then said that she was a bit upset when she left home to come nursing, but a friend of hers looked after him for her. "Who's looking after yours?" she asked.

"A friend of mine," he said.

"Have you seen him lately?" she asked.

"Yes," he replied and burst into tears, "he brought him to see me last week on Wednesday and the dog wouldn't come to me. He didn't seem to want to know me."

Our time was up, we did our best to comfort him, and left for a debrief.

"You can't mend broken hearts with medication," I said. "Come on, let's go and tell the houseman what we've found out."

The houseman was most interested, and talking to the ward sister found out that was the day he stopped progressing. "That's the answer then," he said, "you'd better get that dog back and let him spend some time with him."

I never did find out what happened finally; I did find out that he was discharged home, but with goodwill they would hopefully have brought the two together in hospital, and allowed the healing to be complete. On the debrief of this visit we explored the relationships between persons and animals. I was able to point out that although one is sad and upset by the loss of one's parents – which is inevitable, nobody will live forever – the loss of a friend or lover is different. You choose your friends; there must be something about them that is special or you would not choose them, even a dog, but you are stuck with your parents much as you may love them.

It is a sad fact that stopping and listening for the clues is still not much of a priority in the process of care; the clever people still go on about total patient care, but that's just words and sounds good, and is the right thing to say! But sadly it is often what patients don't say that is ignored, and in that can be the clue to their recovery!

8

THE LEARNING CURVE STEEPENS

With all these extracurricular activities, I was still enjoying my work in nurse education, and at the same time the practice was doing so well I began to wonder if I'd be able to carry on both roles for much longer. I was getting some very good results with my therapy, helping all kinds of patients who had had little help from conventional medicine – and then out of the blue, nemesis struck. The AIDS virus was on the prowl, and after some bright spark in the Ministry of Health produced a brochure advising the general public of the dangers of non-conventional medicine, acupuncture, ear piercing, tatooing etc. carried out at a non-NHS practice. My honeymoon period was brought to an end, and patient numbers dropped from twenty a week to, if I was lucky, four.

The knowledge that I adhered to the association's strict code of practice along with my own knowledge off asepsis – I had taught the subject in the NHS for years – meant nothing. This was written down by a government official, and the pen being mightier than the sword, that held sway! It was a disaster for myself and a lot of other therapists but I was lucky to have my NHS work as well, so we had to sit it out until the hysteria settled. Information and disinformation was churned out, encouraged by the medical profession and newspapers. No acupuncturist had ever spread MRSA – one could not argue that the medical profession were not guilty of that fact, even in centres of excellence, along with hepatitis C, and of course untreated blood which eventually was known to spread the virus of AIDS itself. I spent a lot time with patients advising them that all my needles used were pre-sterilised, and I was an SRN working in the NHS, but it made little difference. I remember one very clever senior officer in the RAF whose wife came to me for treatment, after I had explained this to him he said, "So you say, but can I get AIDS from your needles?"

It was a most frustrating time, and considering that AIDS was spread by infected blood products (it's now screened before use) and by people with alternative sexual appetites, drug abusers and their like, the government of the day did not dare announce this too loudly, for fear of offending a small minority, as it appeared then, of the male adult population.

It took a lot of courage to persevere at that time; so much fuss was being created and so much scaremongering, which sold an awful lot of newspapers and indeed frightened a lot of innocent people, but raised the share prices of the companies producing rubber contraceptives and gloves!

The amount of fuss must have been as great as the vast amount of propaganda produced. Every hospital had to have an AIDS adviser and his assistant. It was incredible to me that the hospitals' own infection control nurses could not cope with this; when I suggested this, I was howled down! However, I was well aware that this was all a potential medical disaster, but as usual, sensationalists as always made the most of it! The extra staff needed must have cost the taxpayer a lot of money.

All this made me look very carefully at a my record keeping. I was quite used to keeping records and had learnt to do this accurately in the RAF. Each promotion course had an element of administration in it; this was a great advantage to me when I started the business, having little trouble in this area. I had been taught how to open files, cross reference and all the thousand-and-one things in good office practice, and now stood me in good stead, but this AIDS scare did shake me out of complacency and make me review what I was doing.

My consulting room, treatment and waiting areas had to be inspected by the environmental health department of the local authority because of the AIDS scare, and were found to be well-run, the comment from the inspector being that I probably knew more about asepsis than he did, which was probably true! So I was sure we would weather this storm eventually. I just had to wait for the hysteria to die down.

One important thing I had learned over the years was how valuable personal contact was when caring for the sick. Initially on meeting a new patient, a handshake was essential to get the relationship off to a good start. But thereafter, to hold the hand of an ill person or someone who is in distress, or lonely, just maybe a touch on the shoulder can work wonders.

This had developed over the years to a sort of gentle massage of either hand or feet as appropriate, but when using acupuncture, which was not necessarily painful, many patients were apprehensive and had suffered enough pain with their condition. I would then say, now the nice bit, I'll massage your shoulders or legs, and they would forget the pain temporarily.

I had learned some of this technique when working in the RAF when in charge of an oncology ward, and now was finding it was quite a powerful adjunct to acupuncture.

I had now been qualified in teaching for over ten years and it was time for me to have another refresher and development course. We were offered a choice of subjects, and I found one at the University of Surrey called therapeutic touch. The university informed me that it was about advanced massage technique. This was a real surprise. I realised that the profession was beginning to haul itself into the present, so I applied and was accepted.

It turned out to be an interesting, well-planned and most informative course with as much practical work as theory, and frankly it showed me another side of myself – all of us have a private bit to our lives, and this uncovered mine for me. I was advised after a couple of days by Carol, the course tutor, to try and stop being the professional therapist, and relax and be myself, to concentrate on just being. This puzzled me at first, but when I did cotton on, I really did become another person, to myself and to my patients. It was very humbling, and what I needed! I now had to change my ways or pay the price!

The course covered the whole spectrum of touch, physical, mental and spiritual. I needed to hone those skills I had and take them to their logical conclusion. It was not what you did, but what you were that counted, and that needed to be on display at all times, in particular when meeting a new, worried patient. It gave me some comfort, in that although I had not done anything wrong, I had often in the past backed off before I should have done, possibly to spare my own feelings.

The university staff, and in particular the tutor Carol, were all very considerate and competent. Carol was a very complete person; I was a bit wary of her for a while after her admonishment to me, kindly said but to-the-point, but thereafter we got on very well together.

Some six weeks later I completed the theoretical part of the course at London University, and received another certificate of competence to add to my growing list of certificates, and so now a degree of authority in what I was doing in this direction was established.

On return from the course, Roy wanted to know what I'd learned, and after an in-depth debrief asked me if I would share my new skills with the student body and the teaching staff.

The subject of therapeutic touch then became an optional extra for all students and I was given a one-day session for each intake, and a number of other hospitals in the group requested my services. It was felt that this gave the ward nurses another skill in the care of the chronic sick, and even the school of midwifery were interested and sent a number of student midwives along to join the fun!

I was now leading a real double life, conventional medicine by day and alternative at evenings and weekends. There was no dichotomy, however, in what I was doing; in fact I felt that I was using the best techniques from both, and practising at a much more sensitive level. Insofar as the massage techniques I'd taught to the nurses, they were now using them when appropriate in the geriatric department, and even giving foot massages to patients in intensive care who were immobile due to therapy or unconscious due to their medical condition. I had noted in the past how even unconscious patients reacted to comforting procedures, shown by slowing of the pulse rate, or the blood pressure reducing slightly; unresponsive a patient might be in most ways, but it is well-documented that an apparently moribund patient has responded to noise or other stimulants.

Certain qualified staff were not keen on nurses 'wasting their time like this' and one staff member was reported to me as having said that I was only teaching the subject so I could get my hands on young nurses! The threat of legal action rapidly put a stop to that nonsense. It was an unpleasant slur and made me feel quite sick. I did wonder how a professional colleague could behave in such a way, and it told me a lot about her.

In my practice I was using more and more massage in combination with acupuncture, and found both therapies worked well together. One patient in particular, a young married woman suffering from Multiple Sclerosis, which had developed after major surgery, came to see me one evening. She was partially paralysed in both legs and could only walk with sticks, and then only a few yards.

She was a small extremely tidy lady, always neatly dressed, and said she used to have an immaculate home, but as she could no longer do the housework, had to stand by as her home deteriorated around her, and this upset her immensely. Because of the spasm in her legs she was always in pain, even when sitting. However, she slept well, but the pain was increasing week by week. This was of course aggravated by the knowledge of her disease and her despair, as she looked at the future, knowing that her condition was progressive. She also had, because of the condition, bladder and bowel problems and needed medicines to relieve these frequently.

All the pills and potions for the spasm and pain had failed to help, she spent a lot of time on her own, her husband was a busy professional man, she had been a civil servant with a good job, and loss of income now was another factor in her life which worried her, so the whole picture was bleak. She had been attending the pain clinic at the hospital, but this provided only some answer to her physical problems – her mental and social problems were not addressed. I was asked by the clinic nurse, an ex-student of mine, if I would see her. The doctor in charge concurred; he was very open minded! I was happy to accept her as a patient.

She came into my office with her husband one evening, a little despairing frightened lady with pain in her eyes. I went slowly through my usual questionnaire and then physically examined her. She now sat before me in my rather comfortable armchair. I moved towards her and took her hands in mine.

"What's the best thing in your life at present?" I asked gently.

"Going to bed at night," she replied quietly.

"And the worst thing?" I asked.

"Waking up in the morning and finding I'm still alive," she said in a low voice. I realised that her horizon was twelve hours; not much of a future in that!

"You do know I can't cure you, don't you?" I said.

"Yes," she knew that, "but can you help the pain?"

"I really don't know, but I'll do my best for you," I replied.

I instituted a regime for easing some of her problems by treating her water works and bowel dysfunction with immediate effect, and massage to her legs and back which after a few days began to relieve some of the pain.

She had cold, wasted legs because of their lack of use, and the massage increased the blood supply to them and so warmed them up. She attended twice a week initially and she began to look forward to the visits; it not only got her out of the house, but she was able to chat about her life both past and present.

One day I asked her if she would come with me to the school of nursing and act as my model for demonstrating massage to the nurses. It would also be of value to them to learn a little about the problems of care for the young disabled and the social and personal problems associated with this type of neurological disease. She agreed to this proposal with alacrity. In the circumstances the hospital would not pay her for her time, I told her, but I promised her a free lunch after each session at a local hostelry, which added to her pleasure and got her back to meeting people again.

These sessions became once a fortnight, and she really began to improve physically and mentally. She felt that for the first time in years she was making a contribution in life as her self-esteem increased.

One day after a few weeks of this regime, I asked her what she was doing for Christmas, and with some enthusiasm she told me that close relatives were coming to stay. Three months previously, she could only see twelve hours ahead, now it was two months. This was a real improvement!

So, after each session she had increased mobility, her bowel and water work difficulties had eased, and life looked a lot better for her. She was much more cheerful and was thinking of others, and was better able to cope with the general attitude of most who dismissed her problems as 'Well you've got MS, what do you expect'. She was also getting more assertive when she was ignored by others, and said to one man who leaned over her in her wheelchair in a shop jumping the queue, "Oi, can't you see me!" He was, she said, quite abashed, and had to apologise.

But all good things have to come to an end. Her husband, on gaining promotion in his profession, was asked to relocate, and she left the city and moved to Norfolk under the tender mercies of the social and medical services, and slowly her condition declined and she lost a lot of what we had achieved over the last eighteen months.

So as I have already said, the treatment of a disease is one thing, but the care that goes with it is equally important.

The school of nursing were also sorry to see her go. She'd become a firm favourite in the department, and had cooperated with other tutors who taught the care of the chronic sick – this being an area in an acute hospital often neglected, as few disabled are admitted with acute problems, and nurses find it difficult to deal with this type of patient unless taught in this area.

About this time the health of my dear mother, now over eighty, was beginning to decline. She lived in a little bungalow in Letchworth. I did my best to visit as often as I could, but was too busy to go as often as I would have liked. The practice was getting busy and the journey down the A1 of some sixty miles was time-consuming.

She had 'gone off her feet' as the saying goes, her home rendered uninhabitable due to a water tank burst, and she had to be taken into Part 3 accommodation until it could be dried out. She was desperately unhappy there, and desperately wanted to get back to her home, but was assessed as being incapable of caring for herself and had to stay in the council-run home.

The staff were very kind to their elderly residents and did their best to make it a home for them, but after a few days mother was admitted to the Lister Hospital in Stevenage in a very low state, and when my brother and I visited that week she was semiconscious and didn't know us. As I was about to leave the ward the staff nurse asked me to see the doctor in charge of her case. I introduced myself and asked him what his plans were for Mother.

He told me he wanted to take her to theatre the following morning to do a biopsy on a lump in her neck. As there was evidence that she was possibly in liver failure this would also need attention.

"Why surgery at her age, what for?" I asked. "For whose benefit, yours or hers?"

He looked startled. "What do you mean?" he asked.

I replied, "She's eighty-nine and a widow and has more and more over the last few years said she wanted to join my father who died in 1949. Also, you would expect somebody of her age to have a number of undiagnosed lumps around, and possibly organ failure. Please leave her alone, keep her comfortable and let her go."

"Well, if that's what you want," he said.

"No, that's not what I want," I replied.

"Well what do you want then?" he asked, looking puzzled.

"I want her back as she was forty years ago, can you do that?" I replied.

"You know we can't," he said.

"So let her go then," I said, then I told him I was a tutor in a geriatric unit and had seen too many people on their last legs whose final days had been made worse by medical intervention. He agreed with me then – I think he was rather relieved – and said they would just keep her comfortable.

I went down again two days later to find she was virtually moribund. I whispered my goodbyes – I hope she heard, as I asked her to give my love to my father when they met again – and got up to go. I went to the desk and told the staff nurse to let me know when she went, and I would contact all the others concerned.

She looked up at me smiled and said, "Are you all right?"

"What do you think?" I said.

She looked at me kindly. That girl was wise beyond her years. She came round the desk, put her arm in mine and said, "Come on, I'll take you to the lift," and without another word escorted me to the lift, whispered goodbye and pressed the button.

As I went down in the lift, I had the strange feeling of going out of my mother's life in a tin box, and then got into another tin box and drove home!

I had to get home, I had a lot of patients to see, but as I finished at 9.30 p.m. the phone rang, and the staff nurse told me that Mother had just slipped away.

My mother, certainly in her own sphere, she was after all born in the Victorian era, subscribed in all ways to those mores. She had not wasted her life; she had made a major contribution to the life of her church, she had a lovely soprano voice and was much in demand as a soloist and choir member, and I remember with much affection the musical evenings we used to have around the piano on a Sunday evening after church.

My two brothers and I had of course spent two years watching her decline into senility and had in effect done our grieving, so it was with a sense of relief that we arranged her funeral. We determined it would be a celebration of her life and we intended it would be so far as was possible, a joyous occasion. And so it turned out to be.

A death in the family causes so much disruption and Mother's death was no exception to the rule. My daughter and granddaughter were staying with Pam and I at the time whilst her husband, who was in the RAF, was away on a course in Nottingham. My younger brother naturally wanted to come to the funeral; he lived in South Wales and would have to travel up and stay with us, so it was arranged that I would pick up my son-in-law in my car as he completed his course on Thursday, before her Friday funeral, and they would all then go home to Norfolk, so making room for my brother Gerald.

I was going to pick him up on Thursday evening at Luton, the terminus of the bus company bringing him up from Wales. So I had a lot of travelling to do, some 300 miles to do in one day, and then my car, only two months old with a small mileage, began to play up, running very roughly and making the most enormous noise from the braking system.

I asked my garage, the main dealer for this make, if they could fit in a quick service on the Thursday morning, and on completion of this drive straight away to pick up my son-in-law at Nottingham.

They duly did this, but as I drove away, the car was no better, just as noisy and running roughly. I was not pleased, but time was of the essence and I had many miles to do.

Still the funeral had to be attended and all the arrangements went ahead to make it as pleasant a time as possible for the very many who wanted to attend. We had been quite careful with our arrangements and made sure that the celebration we had planned went ahead without a hitch.

My younger brother chose the hymns, my elder brother, a professional musician, played the organ, and I read the lesson of my choice. I chose Psalm 59, a psalm she loved – 'How lovely are thy dwellings' – it was an uncomfortable feeling standing next to her coffin on the podium reading, but I wanted to do it well. She was a stickler for everything being done properly, so I did it as well as I could, and think that she would have approved.

On clearing her house before the funeral, among her effects I had found a letter she had written to my father when he was diagnosed with cancer all those years ago. I read the first line and realised this was a love letter and would read no more, so sealed it up well, and before the funeral asked the undertaker to put it into her hand before they screwed the lid on her coffin. There really is so little you can do for the dead, but this gave me satisfaction that I'd done something as a last present for her!

So the funeral came and went, a hole left in our lives which could only be filled with lovely memories, and life returned to normal as we coped with the day to day affairs of living.

However, some weeks later our cat was run over and killed. Pam and I were very upset and shed a few tears; the cat, Zoe we called her for some reason which escapes me, was part of our home and we loved her funny ways. I was possibly more upset with her death that I had been over the death of my mother, and when discussing bereavement with some students in class, told them this. They were appalled that I should have felt this way and accused me of being quite callous.

I reminded them that I had chosen my cat, I didn't chose my mother. Yes, I loved her, but not in the same way as you love things you have chosen, like the death of your child or husband. I told them of my previous occasion with the man and his dog who was not progressing and the students' response to this as they saw it in action.

Your parents, by the natural order of things, will one day die, but the premature death of a dependant that you chose is more shocking in its way.

I remembered this some weeks later when a patient of mine lost his very close friend and business partner. He remarked to me how upset he was at his death, more so than when he had lost his elderly parents some months previously. He found it hard to understand his feelings.

"You choose your friends," I said gently. "He must have been a very special person if you chose him, but you didn't choose your parents, you were stuck with them!"

He thought for a moment, "Yes, you're right," he said, "I hadn't thought of it like that."

Following the funeral I made time to investigate the problems on the car. I found to my astonishment that the sparking plugs, without any check of the spark gap, had been put in as they came out of the pack, and on taking off the brake drums found they were full of asbestos dust from the pads, hence the noise.

I managed to contact the service manager on the Monday morning, who investigated this and returned my call at 1400 hours.

Firstly he apologised about the plugs, and then said, "But we can't do anything about the brakes under health and safety disposal of asbestos regulations."

I stopped him as he got into full flow and said, "You don't know me, do you Mr Green?"

"No sir, I haven't had the pleasure," he replied.

"Well," I said, "you soon will if you give me that load of guff, because you see, I am a lecturer at the hospital and I deal with health and safety, and if you as a company can't deal with asbestos, I will have pleasure in informing the local inspectors who will come and place a prohibition order on you, and close you down until you can cope!"

There was a stunned silence! But of course the outcome of all this was that they did put it right, the next day! I had no more trouble with either the car or the garage.

Thereafter, the poor old garage service staff treated me with a lot more respect, but as I told them, had I been a seventeen-year-old girl they would have got away with their sloppy behaviour, and they felt they had to agree with me! Also did they realise how much of an inconvenience they had put me to in the circumstances?

I really don't know if the HASAW inspectors would have called at my insistence and done their devilish work, but then neither did Mr Green! But it must have frightened the pants off him.

9

LIFE GETS SERIOUS

A few days later I had a call from the College of Acupuncture which initially put me in a bit of a spin. Would I, asked their medical director, give a talk to the annual conference? I was a junior lecturer at the college by now, but this was a great honour. Why me? It so happened that the planned speaker was detained on business in the USA and wouldn't be able to make it. I swallowed, thought, not too deeply, and agreed, but what was the talk to be about?

"Oh," he said, "if you don't want to talk about the things the planned speaker had arranged, whatever you want!"

Well I didn't want to talk about his subject, because I didn't know a lot about it, and the conference was in three weeks' time. I swallowed again, "I'll get back to you in a couple of days," I said hopefully.

I went to bed that night and had a restless troubled night, and then awoke early and suddenly knew what I wanted to say!

Some weeks earlier, I had been asked by the director of the pain clinic at the hospital if I could make time to talk to a pet project of his. It rejoiced under the acronym of SHIP, which stood for 'self help in pain', and to advertise this particular group – the press would be present at the talk. The director was inundated with work, he knew I had a particular interest in treatment of pain, I'd worked in oncology and surgery some years previously and at present in my practice I treated many patients suffering from intractable pain, and knew a lot of the tricks of the trade in this subject.

One of my patients was the chairman of this group, who had chronic pain herself, and I had treated her with some success, so I asked her what she wanted me to say.

"I'll leave that to you," was the helpful reply.

"One thing I can't talk to you about with any authority is pain," I said.

"Why not?" she asked, looking surprised.

"Well I haven't got any," I replied.

She smiled. "Well then, how do you cope with somebody who has?" she asked.

"Ah, that's a different story. The real answer is, with difficulty," I replied.

"Tell us that," then she said, "and we will see what we get out of it!"

It is very harrowing to cope with a person who has intractable pain, and sometimes leaves one with the feeling that you wish you were a mile away when your treatment doesn't always give comfort immediately.

It is quite therapeutic to talk to a well-informed, intelligent patient, and the chairman had a degree in some esoteric subject and was an excellent conversationalist.

I told her some of the problems that many people had when you try and mix alterative with conventional medicine, and of one patient in particular, a young man with severe Hodgkins disease which affected his spinal cord and left him often gasping in pain, which was aggravated by excess vomiting caused by the chemotherapy he was having. His despairing parents brought him to see me as even the anti-emetic drugs he was given did not help, and he had to go thirty miles every two days to the nearest oncology centre for his treatment, and after each treatment he was thoroughly upset and sobbing with pain and vomiting, and his poor parents suffered with him, they were in danger of a breakdown, but nobody had given them much thought. They were watching their dear son dying before their eyes. So I treated him with acupuncture, and after a couple of days got his vomiting under control.

I used a well-known point to insert the needles on the front of the arm above the wrist, and the effect lasted about twenty four hours only, but at least he had relief and the drugs had a chance to work. I had a think about this and decided to try a TENS machine on this point, which he could turn on when he felt nauseated. This worked miraculously, he did not have to see me daily and could come once a week only for a check. The effect on the whole family was obvious; they were beginning to live again.

However, one day he came in looking unhappy. His parents were very annoyed; he'd been told at the oncology centre at the university hospital that the effect of the TENS was a load of nonsense, and it was all in the mind. Poor lad, he had enough to worry about without being told that his vomiting was all his fault!

He continued to decline however, and did eventually sucumb to the disease, but his parents were so grateful that I'd given him some relief as he went along this awful road. After I told this to the chairman she said, "Well there you are then, tell us how you, your patients, and their loved ones can help each other when in pain."

I now went away and had to think long and hard how to help these people who suffered chronic pain. It was no good telling them of my successes, they'd been told often enough, try this or that, this will help, and it did not.

I started off looking for a definition of pain that would be acceptable. All the textbooks talked of pain in various organs, described in detail types of pain, from an ache to indescribable burning lancing pain, but what they did not do was to describe the things that not only exacerbated their existing problems but accompanied them, worry, loneliness, fear, unhappiness, rejection by friends and loved ones and so on. So I came up with definition of my own: 'Pain is an unpleasant sensory experience, with psychological overtones, and social consequences'.

If I was going to talk about being in pain – 'in' is the operative word – I needed a starting point, and this is where I could start.

My audience were a motley crowd; all well-diagnosed, all had lost hope of a cure. I didn't want them to think I could cure them – that would have been thoroughly dishonest and cruel. They were on sticks, in wheelchairs, a couple of amputees and so on. I gave them my definition and explained it to them, pain hurts, they knew that! Pain worried and frightened them, yes they knew that! They'd all lost many friends who didn't see them again, yes they all agreed with that.

So I threw the meeting open, "So what do you do when it gets too difficult, to you, and you, and you?" I asked them, looking round the group, and soon they started talking; one found that so and so helped, somebody else found that something else did and so on. Yes, it was a brotherhood of pain, all in the same boat, now learning from each other how they coped. I couldn't stop them talking! They found they had a lot in common, they were not on their own, the pain they were experiencing was not just physical, it was mental, spiritual, social and so on; and so offered their experiences, and often previously unspoken thoughts and fears, put them all in the pot and realised that others coped somehow. Perhaps they now had some ideas that they could use.

Problems shared bring people together; adversity such as wartime experiences, some of these people remembered this time when all suffered together and somehow got through. So I felt it had achieved something – at least the audience applauded me enthusiastically.

When I phoned back to the director of the conference, I knew I had the bare bones of what I wanted to say. He was most interested and asked for more detail. I told him I would talk about how the patient copes with pain and its many manifestations, how we as practitioners and dealing with intractable pain, how it affects us, and how do the relatives and people who love the patient see it, and try to cope with it.

"Well, we've never done anything like that before," he said.

"No," I replied, "we always talk about treatment, never the person who is in receipt of our ministrations. I'll call the talk 'It hurts doesn't it'!"

He laughed, "That should get the audience's attention," he declared.

So for the next frantic fortnight, I slaved away in all of my very few spare moments, reading all the stuff available from the hospice movements, all books on pain relief, and all of my own notes.

The day of the conference arrived, we all had a good lunch, I purposely avoided any alcohol, and at the appointed time I stood up in front of an audience of some 300 people. Many were of the same peer group as myself, some very experienced and did my thing. I started off with a joke. The audience laughed; they hadn't heard that one before, I was told afterwards, so that was a good start! They continued to laugh at the right bits and looked very thoughtful as I got a bit near the knuckle, but at the end, there was applause and the editor of our professional magazine asked me if I would allow it to go into print. It was therefore rated as a success and worth listening to. Even though I had been very apprehensive at the start, it seemed to flow alright when I got going. Never has an hour gone so quickly!

About six months later I was very flattered to receive a letter from a surgical registrar from a major Peking hospital, saying that he was most impressed with my talk and agreed with all I said. He asked if I would be prepared to host him for a couple of months so he could work in my clinic. That the article had travelled some 8000 miles was amazing, but the man's letter and his request was, in all probability, a means of getting out of China and away from communism, in other words pure politics.

I replied that I did not think that working in my part-time practice where I would see no more than forty patients a week would be any help to a man in a busy city hospital where he would see hundreds, so I told him to write to the dean of the college and ask for his advice. He never did, I was subsequently told, so as I said, it was probably only a means of getting to the West.

10

THINKING OUTSIDE THE BOX

Thinking along more detailed lines since my research into pain responses, I looked more carefully at the painful conditions presented to me in the practice. The pain of loneliness, in loss of friends and loved ones, the pain of humiliation, those who were not believed when they were ill and needed help and were treated with little sensitivity for their feelings. The pain of degrading treatments carried out with little respect for the patient's sexuality.

So many of my patients had many disparate problems and had been abandoned by their medics and told to stop wasting the NHS's time or to 'learn to live with it'. The tests show nothing amiss so there is nothing wrong with you!

On the reply, 'Well why don't I feel well then' the usual response had been a shrug of the shoulders or some other indication that they were time-wasters or attention-seekers. So keep taking the tablets!

So far as I was concerned, we all need attention of some sort even when well, but to deny this to the sick was a denial of their very humanity. The pain of rejection, of the outcast, leads one to seek attention by fair means or foul. Kids do it by screaming, teenagers by getting into trouble with the authorities and adults, sadly having been brought up to the stiff-upper-lip approach to life, have to suffer alone.

To me, the fact that somebody feels he needs attention shows that person has something wrong, in that his basic needs are not being met, and unless he can be shown that he is mistaken, and there is a reason for his pain, then listening carefully is the best way to deal with him. Listening, not just hearing, and listening for the clues – they are all there somewhere. It's not a waste of time, letting the patient talk; for them it can be very therapeutic even if it bores the pants off you. 'A burden shared' etc. is wisdom indeed.

Insofar as the person who has been told to learn to live with it, I always ask, 'Have you been offered any teaching?' If you have to learn, you need a teacher! Unfortunately, it is rare that they have been offered.

One young woman came to see me, she was totally demoralised. She had ulcerative colitis and for two years had been living in a Commonwealth country with her husband, who was an engineer of some standing in the profession. She had only reluctantly joined her husband as he had a three-year government posting, and she was pregnant when she went.

She had the baby, which was a stressful enough time, being away from friends and relatives, and developed the disease after the birth. She had a number of close relatives at home who suffered bowel disease but never thought she would develop it. However, she was miles away from medical help; the nearest hospital was staffed by expatriate Eastern Europeans who had little sympathy for women, and English ones at that, and all investigations and treatments were done with little or any consideration for her feelings. Also at the end of the initial treatment, the bill was so colossal that they had to return to UK or go bankrupt.

By this time she was having some twenty-four bowel actions daily and was down to five-and-a-half-stone in weight. On arrival back in the UK, she was cared for by the local consultant, but her mental state now was so low she did not respond to treatment. Her consultant, a man I knew well and had a lot of respect for, was very worried, and after a week or so told her the only answer to this was major surgery to remove the diseased bowel. She felt that this was too much to bear. He said to her in desperation, "If you don't have it done, it will go cancerous and you will die."

When first she saw me, she told me what he said. "I knew that deep down, but I didn't need to be told like that!" she stated.

My first objective was to comfort her and then try and stop the diarrhoea. She was past counselling, she would hear nothing, she was so withdrawn into herself. I used acupuncture points to stop the diarrhoea, made her warm and comfortable on my couch, wrapped her in a blanket, and began to massage her feet with oil. I put some quiet music on the tape machine and kept her there for an hour. This was the pattern of treatment for six weeks, and slowly the tension ebbed away, she started to put on weight and the diarrhoea slowed to twice a day. This lady really needed somebody on her side, I wrote in her notes, 'this lady needs a friend, what a pity she has to buy friendship!'

She appreciated straight talking, and on her tenth visit she gaily waltzed into the clinic looking so much better. "Well," I said, "you look good, what do you want to ask me?"

She laughed, "How do you know I want to ask you something? But you're right," and she said mischievously, "if you are so clever, what do I want to ask you?"

"The question, Jane, is, 'I feel so well, do I need the operation?' And the answer is yes, you're forty now, and I'm getting on for sixty and won't be around for ever. You need an answer to your problem and so far as I know, surgery is best for you."

She had been referred to the gastroenterologist, and he had agreed that she needed surgery, but it was so complex an operation, she was advised it would take at least three months to get organised and get the team together if she wanted to proceed.

This worried Jane; she had agreed to go ahead with it, but found the wait would be unbearable if she was given a proposed date for the surgery weeks ahead.

I asked her if she would like me to ask the administration to hold the information until a couple of days before the surgery was to take place, and they could then contact her husband, tell him the date, and the day before he could tell her and she would then go straight in for the preparation which itself would take a couple of days.

She thought this was a wonderful idea, so I arranged it for her and she then got on with her life, still seeing me weekly, and by now was feeling very well indeed. However, the well-laid plans of mice and men of course went awry, and as usual in an organisation as big as the NHS, somebody did not communicate with someone else, and two months before the surgery, they phoned her and not her husband and gave her the date! So she had a bad couple of months which undid some of the progress she had made. But things did work out eventually; she had the surgery, it was extensive and required three separate surgical sessions, and after a long stay, she returned home to recuperate with my help.

Some two years later I saw her out shopping and she looking very well. I asked her if she could recall her first visits to me and what it did for her.

She said that when I massaged her feet it felt as if I was charging her batteries up, and without that she could not have progressed as she did. It seems to be quite amazing how you can transfer energy to another person by touch, and maybe that is why physical therapies are often so exhausting to give. I recall that with Jane that at the end of the first sessions I used to be quite worn out – she'd taken all my energy! So much for massage then, I thought, so I had been right about it all the time! The operation certainly saved her life and sanity, and I like to think that I had a major role in her return to health. Doubtless the medical authorities would not agree to that premise, but I am satisfied that my care was right for her at that time in her life when she could see no future.

Being still on the hospital's tutorial staff, I was often able to stand to one side and even indirectly influence events. It didn't always work out, as in Jane's case, but that wasn't my fault.

One afternoon I came across a young nurse who was 'specialing' an elderly, confused patient. The term meant that one special nurse was detailed to look after a patient who had special needs, and in this case, in spite of treatment and some sedation, this patient was irrational, very restless and needed continual observation.

"What's the reason for her state?" I asked her, recognising a teaching situation.

"She's confused," she replied.

"Yes, I can see that," I said, "but why is she so?"

"I don't know," she said.

"Well, we'd better find out, go and get me her notes," I replied.

The girl brought them back. They were not a lot of help, only reporting that she had been confused so they had put this usually ambulant woman to bed, and she had fallen out once, but no damage had been done.

She was suspected of having a chest infection and had been prescribed antibiotics, but the staff found it difficult to get her to take them. I took her pulse, which was weak and rapid, and felt her skin, which was hot and dry, and opened her mouth; it was so dry they had no chance of getting pills into this eighty-year-old lady! She was extremely dehydrated.

I asked to see her fluid output chart. She had not passed any urine, nor had she drunk anything for twenty-four hours.

"Well there's the answer," I said, "why isn't she drinking?"

"She won't drink anything, we try to give her a cup of tea but she shakes her head," she replied.

"Let me look at her notes again," I said, and on her admission a few weeks ago, in a section called personal preferences it was written, 'Does not like tea or coffee'. "Well there's the answer," I said. "That's why she won't drink, so what have you given her then?" I asked.

"She won't drink anything!" Back to square one!

The patient was semi-conscious but I put my mouth to her ear and asked, "What would you like to drink my dear?"

She whispered, "I'd love some iced water."

"There you are," I said to the nurse, "take a jug into the kitchen and get some."

She came back and said there were no ice cubes in the fridge. I sent to three other wards in this brand new unit, but no ice trays had been issued with the fridges on commissioning! So I went down to the main kitchen got some ice, took it back and gave the poor woman a few sips of iced water. She was so grateful; she was Irish, and whispered that it was like water from the Liffey!

I then told the nurse to give her half a cup every half an hour until she started to pass water. Four hours later I was told she was responding to treatment. I then went up to the office of the nursing officer of the department.

"Hello, what do you want?" he asked.

"Do you want to save some money?" I asked him.

"You bet," he said, "why do you ask?"

"You'll have to spend to do it."

"We've got orders to spend nothing, this new department has cost an arm and a leg," he said.

"A quid," I said, "for two ice trays in the fridge," and told him about the dehydrated patient. "You've got a girl sitting there doing nothing when she could be doing something useful, you're wasting money. Money is to be used, not wasted." He wouldn't budge, he'd been told not to spend money and that was that. A typical tick-box mentality, a trait that was becoming more and more the norm, I had noticed, in the NHS, this sense of not having the correct priorities!

Another area in which I was becoming interested was the patient's own perception of priorities, often referred to as the 'by the way syndrome' – that is, after all the treatment is over and the patient is satisfied that you have worked the miracle or whatever, as they turn to go, say 'Oh by the way, can you do…' something for whatever else is troubling them but up to now had not been mentioned. This sometimes turns out to be a greater problem than the problem of which they originally complained.

One young woman complained of lower back pain and felt she was walking sideways at times. The pain had proved to be resistant to some three months' conventional physio and analgaesics. She asked for my help. She stated that she was quite fit otherwise, but did not look well. I had seen her before socially and knew her quite well, and we discussed family matters and holidays and so on. As an acupuncture practitioner one has more time to deal with a patient than general practitioners, so often both can learn a lot of facts from each other.

It was a cold winter's day and we commented on this, and I remember telling her that in my childhood we were often cold, particularly at night when the fire was put out, and often awoke in the morning to ice on the widows and in the kitchen sink and so on. No central heating in those days!

I observed that this was often the cause of a lot of chest and throat infections in the days prior to antibiotics, and earache was quite a common complaint among children causing a lot of distress. I recalled an episode when I had a 'runny ear' and a stiff neck, and a lot of kids started like this and ended up with mastoiditis and needed surgery.

"Oh," she said. "That's what my doctor thought I could have some months ago."

"Did he treat you?" I asked.

"Yes, he gave me some pills and it seemed to settle it down, anyway, I've got to go now, I've got a hair appointment."

The conversation ended. We arranged another appointment to see her in a few days. With that she eased herself out of the chair. Her back was now less stiff, but as she stood up to go, she had to put out her hand to me to steady herself. She said, "By the way, I'm quite dizzy at times."

"Sit down again," I said, reaching for my auroscope. There it was, a bulging ear drum! Hence the dizziness; the antibiotics obviously didn't clear the infection, so I treated her with a decongestant treatment and inhalations, and when she came back next week she said the dizziness had gone and she was now walking straight again – she hadn't realised she had been walking differently – and also the back ache had disappeared!

"Well, what do you know," she said laughing, "never thought a bad ear could make your back ache!"

Another elderly lady came to see me with what she said she had been told was lumbago. On examination I found that she had strained her sacro-iliac joints pulling up weeds in the garden. She was over eighty and loved pottering in her cottage garden, watched as a rule by her demented husband; he seemed to get pleasure just watching her work.

She found the gardening a welcome relief from watching over poor old George, but was now quite distressed that she found it difficult to bend to her task. I treated the back successfully for a couple of weeks, for which she was most grateful, and as she was about to go I got the 'by the way' again.

"What is it Ruby?" I asked.

"I've got a lump, Mr Donald," – she always called me that.

"Come on Ruby," I said, "come back and sit down. Where's the lump, in your boob?" I asked her.

She showed me, a nasty fungating late-stage carcinoma leaking all over her bra.

"How long have you had this?" I asked.

"About a year," she replied.

"You know what it is?" I asked.

Yes, she'd guessed it was cancer, but was worried about George and what would happen to him if she went into hospital.

"It's got to be dealt with," I said and wrote a note to her GP, and within a fortnight she was in hospital and had a total mastectomy.

I went to see her in hospital. She looked very well and was the pet of all the staff; they loved her cheerful demeanour.

"They're looking after me so well," she said beaming, "and I've learnt something since I've been in here."

"And what's that"? I asked.

She replied, "I didn't think much of coloured folks up to now, but these coloured girls are wonderful."

"Well that's a lesson well learned," I said, "what about your operation?"

She looked me straight in the eye and said very seriously, "I'm not sure, I'm only half a woman now with only one."

I often told the nurses this story; so often the youngsters working in geriatric medicine felt that age and sexuality were two different things, and that state of mind gives us mixed-sex wards, which cause a lot of distress to the elderly, and still happens irrespective of what our clever politicians may say about their abolition.

I was teaching some nurses new to the department about the language elderly people may use when talking about their bodily functions. One very well-bred young lady was timorously questioning a deaf old lady about her bowel actions; she was most embarrassed doing this. The old dear shouted back, "What do you mean by me bowels girl, bugger me bowels, I want a man!"

Never a dull moment on the geriatric wards!

One of the ambulance drivers who was well-known to the patients, as he often ferried them to other departments for treatments and so on, spoke to me one day in the corridor. He was looking rather green about the gills.

"What's up with you Jim?" I asked him.

"Mrs Plumpton, bed five," he said, almost gagging.

"What about her," I asked.

"She gave me some peeled brazil nuts last week," he said.

I laughed, "And you took them? Never do that, you don't know where they've been."

"Quite so," he said, "and I enjoyed them, but she told me today that she'd got some more for me when she'd sucked the chocolate off them!"

"Never accept anything unwrapped, especially if it's brown!" As I said, never a dull moment, but a hard lesson to learn!

11

GETTING THE MESSAGE ACROSS

The double life I was leading continued, and as my work in my practice increased so did my work in the school of nursing. I was getting on to sixty years old, and although thoroughly enjoying both roles, it was tiring, and once or twice Pam had to wake me up when I went to sleep in the bath at night!

We began to be a little more aggressive in our approach to recruiting, spreading our search for suitable candidates from the senior schools in the area. As the local careers teachers at the various schools seemed to have little knowledge of the nursing profession as a career, the director asked me to put a presentation together for these people, informing them of the origins, its place in society now and future developments. This was put to an invited audience of teachers who were fortunately impressed with my efforts, and asked a lot of questions. I used different officers in various departments and roles also to speak, and from this we progressed to inviting whole years of fourth and fifth-year students to come and have a taster for an afternoon. These sessions proved to be most popular, and we began to get more applications, and therefore were able to select more suitable students.

Each taster session usually involved some twenty students, each to some ten different seminars of short duration dealing with specific topics. Every ten to fifteen minutes they changed to another session; this gave them a lot of informed opinion, and made many of my colleagues work their socks off. Most admitted to me at the end of an afternoon that they were exhausted talking about the same subject to ten groups for four hours! But the system worked and a good time was had by all.

We did it in all some four times, but that was enough for one year, as we had covered most if not all of the secondary schools in the area.

We were also having management courses for senior staff who wanted to progress. I had done management courses in the RAF, and with a degree of adjustment was now involved in some aspects of these.

It was at the time of the government's idea of the patients' charter, which was sent to individual training and teaching hospitals for local teams to adapt general principles to their own situation.

There was much discussion about this; some were all for it, others felt, 'what do they know about it and why is the government interfering in hospitals anyway?' and so on. 'Surely we know what's best for our patients!' However, this rather negative response, in my view, precluded any informed discussion, and no opinions could be arrived at sensibly unless we did discuss what we were doing. The 'we've always done it this way' brigade were having a ball.

The waiting lists for high tech treatments was growing. We couldn't go on like this much longer; the usual government response up to this time was just to throw money at the NHS, but it was becoming apparent that a new way of running affairs was needed. It seemed that there was – and indeed still is – an idea that the NHS could be run as a business, but failed to recognise that it was not a profit-making organisation, but was a labour-intensive organisation which had to be paid for, but run economically.

A rethink was needed to bring it up to date, but the changes that needed to be considered were to be thoughtful, not knee-jerk reactions.

This was a good time to introduce these thoughts into the management courses then being run.

One day it was my job to introduce a new course to a group of line managers, ward sisters, midwives and physiotherapists. The problem with these people was that most had been promoted to their posts by time qualification only, often to fill gaps in the workforce, and of course they'd learned their role from their predecessors who were of the old school and had passed on a lot of the bad habits, which to them were the norm.

So we had some pretty entrenched attitudes, and at least half of them didn't think they should be there on the course – although all were volunteers – and were at times quite hostile to think that education staff knew anything about the coal face, where did we live then, in ivory towers etc.? As the news of the new patients' charter had just been announced, I mentioned this in my introduction; there was immediately a buzz of comment.

One of the more mature students said loudly, "What a load of rubbish. We can't do anything like that, what do they know about it?"

There was general agreement about this so I let them moan a bit and then called the class to order.

"Right," I said after a minute or so, "how many of you applied for this course?" They all had, nobody had been seconded to it, so after some discussion about applying for courses and courses available for promotion purposes I went on. "Who do you think, coming back to this charter you all seem to dislike so much, suggested it?

"Oh, some idiot in management," one replied. "They're all the same, that lot."

"Really, the same group that you hope to join when you finish here next week?" I said with a raised eyebrow. "So you want to join the idiots?"

There was silence at this. My introduction continued; I told them we would also be talking about various aspects of the law as applied to the medical professions as well as criminal law, and in general concerning the ability of local authorities to make by laws as a matter of interest. It was also the time when the poll tax was being given an airing.

At this one of the class started to laugh and nudged her neighbour who pushed her away.

"Come on," I said, "What's the joke?"

The one who had laughed said, "My friend won't be paying that."

I turned to the one concerned and asked her why.

"I don't agree with it," she said.

I replied, "There's lots of things I don't agree with, but we have to conform in a democratic society."

She laughed, "Maybe, but I'm still not paying it. I've not got a house or kids at school, don't drive a car, so I don't see why I should be taxed on a room I rent from the hospital."

"So what are you going to do if the council insist that you pay it? They may well prosecute you and demand the money, or else!"

"I still won't pay it," she laughed.

"They will take you to court, you will be fined," I said.

"And I won't pay that either in the circumstances," she replied.

"You will be then in contempt of court and may be sent to prison," I informed her.

"So what," she replied, "people who don't pay only get about two weeks in prison, it says so in the papers."

"And you would go to prison on a matter of principle?" I asked.

"Yes," she replied, laughing.

"What will you do when you come out?" I asked seriously.

"Go back to work of course," she said.

"Yes I'm sure you would, but as what?" I asked her.

"I'm a midwife," she replied.

"No you are not," I said, "you are now a criminal with a record and will probably be struck off," she looked shocked.

"Come on," she said, "that's not fair!"

"No, what's not fair is that I have to listen to your childish response to this. If you cannot obey a simple law like that, how can we trust you to comply with the medicine act and controlled drug legislation?"

I was often surprised at the narrowness of vision of so many nurses, who were after all supposed to be accountable and responsible members of a profession.

The other area of legislation I was tasked with teaching was the Health and Safety at Work Act. As safety representative for the school of nursing, and as previously stated, I had done a number of courses on the subject, it fell to my lot to organise various seminars, and also to attend and to take part in the hospital safety committee meetings, also to organise teaching sessions for all grades of staff and tradesmen employed by the hospital.

To do this I had to liase with the fire officers, safety officer and other senior administrative staff, this really broadened my perception of what was really going on in a busy hospital. It's like a small town, with hundreds of trades and professions working in it. Quite an eye-opener to get such an overview, but like a lot of big organisations, the problem is getting each section to talk or understand each other.

I was asked by the electricians, for example, to talk about electrical safety – what did I know about that? They expected me to, however, so I had to find an expert somewhere to do the honours, and others wanted other information, and so I became quite expert in finding people who did know something about it, but of course, hospital electrics, for example, are not the same as in industry or retail businesses. But I learned as I went along, and quite fascinating I found it to be.

I couldn't have done too bad a job, however, as the administration were impressed by the efforts of the school of nursing and we earned a lot of brownie points for what we were doing. Having been brought up as it were in the RAF, problems were settled there on a friendly basis between departments because otherwise chaos resulted and nothing got done. But as I had discovered to my chagrin, NHS cooperation within the hospital was a rare thing! However, I did learn a lot about industrial relations, and when the porters went on strike, they couldn't have cared less that the patients in the hospital were indirectly inconvenienced in some way, even though I observed that there could be trouble if other staff, deputising for them and not qualified to do their job, caused an accident.

This was just met with a shrug of the shoulders. It was the management's fault, they declared. How many times did I hear that remark! Had they never heard of responsibility?

Apart from all my many extracurricular activities, I was still involved with nurse training in areas colleagues didn't feel comfortable in dealing with, in particular when dealing with ethical concepts of care.

We'd already had the acceptance of abortion, and in the future, the concept of 'assisted death' was on the cards; we knew that years ago before it hit the public domain, and were well aware of it, in its modified form it has turned into the Liverpool Pathway! But the hospital chaplains were often asked to talk about these subjects, with the predictable response from the nurses who, being essentially practical people, couldn't get their mind round such profound thinking, and needed the facts put into a more physical and recognisable scenario.

At this time in the late 1980s we were still training rather than educating, and although we were turning out good nurses, the idea that they should be more reflective in what they were doing was a foreign country. But of course, one's own ethical concept relied upon upbringing in the home, parental belief and influence, and of course our students of this time were the children of the sixties, of the Beatles and other external influences upon their morality, and we were asking them to deal compassionately with the lost, the dying, the lonely and those coming towards the end of this life's journey, so a different approach was needed.

An attitude that you could do your own thing irrespective of who suffered was a problem, it seemed at that time we were becoming a very selfish nation.

One afternoon I took a session with a group of senior students, all within a month of becoming registered. This session was billed as 'on accountability and responsibility in nursing'. In line with my line of thinking, I used the critical incident approach much favoured by the American educationists after the war to train returning servicemen to civilian life when their education had been spoiled by hostilities.

The scene I painted for them was of a busy surgical ward on the evening of operating day. There were six post-op patients, three of them still semi-conscious, one who was needing frequent observations as he was thought to be at risk of kidney failure. To cope with this ward were a total of four staff, the staff nurse in charge, two student nurses, one first-year and the other second-year, and one auxiliary who spoke poor English.

The staff nurse had asked for another trained nurse to keep her eye on the very sick patient, but had been told there were no extra staff available because of a high sickness rate of gastroenteritis among the staff that evening. I asked the students if they recognised the scene.

"Oh yes, happens all the time," they replied.

So said I, "This scene is potentially explosive should one staff go sick, do you not agree?"

"Yes, that is so," they replied.

"Should it be allowed to happen?" Certainly not was the general response. There should always be enough staff. But unfortunately, in the scene I described, just before the ward was opened for visitor the staff nurse was rung by A and E and told that her daughter aged five had been brought in with a broken leg having been knocked down by a hit-and-run driver. Her husband was there and wanted her to come down to A and E immediately because he was very shocked at what had happened, he'd only turned his back on her for a second and she'd run into the road. Her injury however was not life threatening. What should she do?

Go and discuss this, I said, and bring me the answer in five minutes!

When they returned the class was split 75/25 in favour of the staff nurse going to her daughter.

This was now discussed quite hotly by those who disagreed! So I asked them then, "Where did the staff nurse's duty lay and to whom?"

So we now came to the concept of management and assessment of risk and professional responsibility. I still had not finished with them!

Sadly one of the class had been killed in an RTA whilst driving home one evening from hospital few weeks ago. After all the fuss had died down and the post mortem held, the class attended her funeral at Leicester crematorium.

"Why did you go?" I asked. The students were a little upset at this question, but we were dealing with matters of life and death, and I thought they were mature enough at the age of twenty-one to discuss this. There was no reply to this. "So," I said. "Well let me give you some reasons and see if any apply. You went as part of your own grieving process for a dear friend, you went to support the family in their loss, you went for a skive" – this really annoyed them, but I ploughed on – "you went as a student body to show you mourned a dear friend as a joint expression of solidarity which helped you all at that sad time?" There were a few rumblings of disquiet as I enumerated those reasons.

"So who gave you permission to be away from the hospital for an afternoon and to be paid for it?" I asked.

"Sue, our own tutor," they replied.

"No, she has no power to do that or authority, so who was it?" I asked.

"Must have been the director," they replied.

"Yes, it was he," I said, "and did he go too?"

"Yes, he was with us," they replied.

"Now then," I said, "what would have happened if whilst you were away there had been a bad train crash at the station with a lot of dead and injured, and it was every possible nurse had to be on duty and you were not there, but fifty miles away?"

"That's not very likely," they observed.

"No," I replied, "the Titanic only sank once, but at the subsequent enquiry, who would have been the one standing before them and admitting that he'd been at a funeral? It would have been the director. You can imagine what the head of the enquiry would have said, 'At a funeral, Mr Director, why? You mean that you took twenty-five pairs of nursing hands to a funeral. In hospital time? Come now. Surely Mr Director, your job is to look after the living, not to bury the dead!'

"And when the boss decided to go, and gave you permission to go, he had to do a risk assessment, and if he had been wrong, it would have been his head on the block, not yours! And that is why he is paid so much more than you, and when you qualify next month, and your salary goes up by one third; even though you will still be doing the same job you've been trained for, you will be paid for making important decisions too, and be responsible for their outcome! That's known as accountability, so think again about the staff nurse and her injured daughter."

A rather subdued student body left the room. I hope they got the message!

Another task that I was landed with was to teach the drug course. This was a semi-practical course to reinforce to the staff the importance not of only knowing the dose and effect of the medication prescribed by the medical staff, but the legal background of the various acts of parliament concerned with the storage, use and therapeutic values of the many preparations on the prescribers' list, which seemed to change daily. The many drug companies that produced medication were from all corners of the globe, and the drugs had to be licensed for use, but many used either their own company name, the chemical name, or a fancy name made up by the producer to have some relation to what the drug was used for. So to a lot of nurses it was a nightmare to remember all these names, as indeed it was to the pharmacists, and each consultant had his favourite ones which he preferred to prescribe that probably differed from his colleagues'. The drug may well have had the same pharmaceutical action, but a different name. Many an elderly patient would come into hospital with up to twelve different prescribed drugs. For example, the patient had been vomiting due to an unintended overdose of a common painkiller, as they called it, and had been prescribed an anti-emetic drug, which had made them sleepy, and as they couldn't get up out of bed frequently became constipated, which was then treated with a laxative preparation which gave them diarrhoea, which caused them to lie in a soiled bed, so they developed a pressure sore, which became infected so were given an anti-biotic, which gave them a skin rash! Many elderly had been seen by various medics in the community, never the same one twice, so the drug schedule had not been modified or stopped when it had done its job and many elderly patients kept boxes of unused drugs and used them as they saw fit for other reasons, or even gave them to fellow sufferers for reasons unbeknown to medicine! It could be a nightmare!

This sounds an unlikely scenario in a modern society, but it does happen and nurses needed to be aware of this, so it fell to me on the course to help the nurses to understand the problem in our society that 'there is a pill for every ill' concept.

Not only this, but the cost of some of these drugs was quite excessive when compared with their intended effect, the drug bill at the hospital increased year on year and was giving concern to the administration, and it was quite possible with a good knowledge of the list of approved medicines, to find alternative ones that had the same or equivalent effect. The doses of the drugs changed frequently; this increased the drug companies' profits but did not necessarily have any beneficial effect for the patient. The administration therefore had to do something about it, so the Drugs and Therapeutic Substances Committee was formed to deal with this.

It consisted of two consultants, a senior nursing officer, the chief pharmacist and myself as the representative from the school of nursing. We were expected to take an overview of where the money was being spent and on what, and either stop their use, or find and recommend an alternative.

On the first meeting I attended, the pharmacist wanted to know why we were using Sterets in such a large number. It had cost £2000 the previous year using these small pre-packed, spirit-soaked swabs to clean the skin prior to the administration of injections. The question was debated, and it was found that very rarely were injections used for drug administration today. Drugs today were mostly taken by mouth, so why were injection swabs being used?

I was asked if I had any idea, and replied that I had seen them used to clean spectacles, to wipe up spills, clean thermometers, I had even seen staff clean the mirrors on their cars with them, but rarely, apart from in ITU or the operating theatre, had I seen them used for injections.

One of the consultants then said that he had told the nurses on his ward not to use them to clean the skin prior to giving an injection of insulin to his diabetic patients, as it made the skin tough for future injections, but the other consultant was unworried about this.

I pointed out that it was the written hospital policy to use them, prior to giving injections, although modern research showed it to be an unnecessary action so long as the skin was socially clean. So to prevent any confusion, if a patient developed a skin abscess, and the nurse was accused of using the incorrect aseptic technique of not using the swabs, and she was disciplined, would he kindly write to the hospital infection committee who wrote the instructions for the authority, and inform them of his wishes, because as I pointed out, it's always the one at the bottom of the heap who gets the blame when things go wrong. So he agreed to this, and our bill for Sterrets virtually disappeared!

12

HELPING THE LOST!

Another role I was expected to perform as part of my teaching role was to give pastoral care to young students often attempting to swim in the sea of an adult world, and to keep their heads above water.

Many a youngster would take the word of some senior staff as gospel without knowing how to recognise that the old one of 'that's how we always do it, so don't argue' was not only wrong but personally dangerous, and in their private lives they were open to abuse due to their own inexperience.

One senior student told me one day in passing that as her car was out of action she was not able to get home to her brother's birthday. I asked her if her car was damaged. She said one of the physiotherapist managers had hit it in the car park and the steering was damaged, and she could not afford to get it repaired because it would cost more than the car was worth, a common problem of relative values for students the world over!

"Well, claim on your insurance," I said.

"I can't," she said, "the physio said that as the accident happened on private property it was invalid."

I laughed, "And you believed her?" I said, "well go and get details of her insurance, and if she won't give them to you, tell the police that she refused, and they can charge her with failing to report an accident, failing to exchange insurance details, and also let your insurance know all about it!" Which of course she did, and got the car repaired.

This was most improper behaviour of one professional to another, by a person who should have known better.

One morning three students came to see me in some distress. They'd held a party the night before in the recreation room but it had been gatecrashed, they claimed, by some youths from the town who had wrecked the place, put broken glass and urinated in the swimming pool, and also abused the home warden.

These three were hauled in front of the accommodation officer. They were banned from partying for six months, and they were to be charged £2000 for repairs and an undisclosed sum for emptying and refilling the pool!

With the innocence of youth they thought it wasn't fair, how could they pay that huge sum?

"Did you get permission to hold the party in the first place?" I asked.

"Oh yes, we had to fill in a form," the spokesman replied.

"What did it say?" I asked.

"We don't remember!"

"Did you read it before you signed it?" Silence greeted this question! "You'd better get me one of these forms and let me have a look at it," I went on, "and you can't afford to pay for the repairs I assume, can your parents?"

"No, our parents will kill us."

"Not surprised," I replied. "Never fill in a form until you know what the implications are for you."

The form they brought back to me was a small sheet of A5 stating that if they were given permission, any damages to the property would have to be paid for in full, and that those attending would have to be named.

I laughed, "I don't think that would hold up in a court of law, who signed it?"

"We all did."

"Did you advertise the party?"

They replied, "No, we were told not to."

"How did the yobs know then?"

"Well, we may have put a little notice in the hall."

"And the hall is a public right of way!" I observed.

"We didn't know that!" they replied.

"Well it is," I informed them, "and there are a lot of predators sniffing around nurses' homes, believe me, and one of them read it, and told his friends. So what do you intend to do, pay up?"

"We can't," they wailed, "our parents will be furious, what are we going to do?"

"You wait here," I said, "and I'll go and talk to the man himself."

The accomodation officer was a new appointee, older than myself, and happened to be ex-RAF. I introduced myself and we got on like a house on fire; he was a bit fed up with some of the funny ways of the NHS, and we compared notes. "If they'd burnt the place down and it cost millions, according to that chit they'd have to pay it all. Not very likely is it?" I told him. He agreed to this assumption.

"What about the three?" I asked.

"I'll have to think about it," he said.

"Will you let me deal with it?" I asked.

"Willingly," he replied, laughing.

"They will be a bit more careful after this!" I said. "They need to be made aware of the seriousness of their position."

"OK, you deal with them then." I went back to them; they looked a bit green about the gills as if they were waiting for their executioner!

"Right you three," I started, "I've seen the boss, you've got three choices. One, you can brazen it out and threaten him with a solicitor."

"We can't afford that," they cried.

"Two, you can offer to pay a fixed sum out of your salary for the next few years."

"We'll be working for next to nothing," they bleated.

"True, or three, you can grovel and say you're very sorry, didn't realise you'd done something stupid and that you've learnt your lesson and won't do it again," I said.

"We're not doing that," they declared, "who does he think he is?"

"You'll find out if you aren't careful! Think about it, I'll be back in five minutes," I said and left the room.

I went back five minutes later, the older one of the three said, "If we apologise and admit to it all will he let us off?" She at least was showing a bit of sense.

"That's the risk you've got to take," I replied. "You've got to take the responsibility on your own shoulders."

"OK then, we'll grovel," they said, "if you will come with us."

So I paraded them in front of the accommodation officer and their spokeswoman said her piece.

He told them off and said don't let it happen again, gave them a few words of advice, and also told them he would rescind the six month ban and make it a month. He also told them that the form they signed would be rewritten to make legal sense and told them to get back to work.

Helping the Lost!

He thanked me for my help and agreed that security of the nurses' home needed to be reviewed as a matter of urgency. The three girls left, and I heard them chattering with relief as they went off down the corridor into the nurses' home, and as I left, I passed the warden's office. She called me in as she was having a cup of tea with the catering officer.

"Were they the three of your nurses who caused all the trouble last night?" she asked.

"Our nurses," I corrected her.

"Yes, of course," she replied. "Well, they were laughing," she said.

"Is there a law against laughing then?" I asked. "Is that hospital policy?"

"I thought nurses were supposed to be responsible people," said the caterer.

"They are," I said, "a lot more responsible than you when you went on strike last year and none of the patients or staff had a hot meal for five days," and walked out. She never spoke to me again!

Yes, these young girls were vulnerable, and often I had to act as their advocate when they had done something thoughtless.

At one of our smaller hospitals in the authority we used to send our pupils and students for special experience, such as learning to cope with children who had, as it is now termed, learning difficulties, that is those children who were incapable of doing the most simple tasks. This was of great value to these nurses in that when these children were admitted to an acute hospital, it was sometimes with great difficulty that they were able to get the attention they deserved, because of the failure of these poor kids to realise the need for other and sick patients to get peace and quiet, and it was essential that they taught them to use toilets properly and leave them unsoiled for the other patients. Many nurses did not like the experience at this hospital and felt threatened, so needed a shoulder to cry on when it became too much for them. Bizarre behaviour is quite upsetting when first one comes into contact with it, but it was of great value to the students to learn how to cope with this type of patient.

The senior staff at these units were well-trained in the care of disabled young patients, and did their best to accommodate these students, but it was sometimes a bit difficult for them to remember their own first experiences in their youth working with these often disturbed patients.

I can recall one youngster who gave the wrong drug to one of these patients, and was hauled over the coals and told there could be a case against her.

I went to see her and investigated the incident as quickly as possible, and found that at the time she was not being supervised by a member of the trained staff; the person concerned was busy doing something else and told the nurse to hand out a prescribed drug, and she gave it to the wrong patient – the patient, of course, had no understanding of what was going on – a very irresponsible thing to do, to allow a trainee to give out drugs without supervision. The culprit eventually admitted it was her own fault, but not before the innocent nurse had had nightmares about it and had been told by others, who should have known better, that she could face dismissal. However, as I told her, it was a lesson well learned for both her and the staff nurse, who was severely reprimanded.

Bullying appeared to be endemic in the NHS and proliferating. Before the NHS the matron and ward sisters ruled the roost, were very professional and knew how to handle people. But the new generation of managers did not appear to consider themselves accountable and would look for the weakest staff member they could accuse of supposed wrongdoing onto whom to shift the blame, and even threaten them with dismissal, although they themselves had no authority to interfere with a nurse's contract, and no power of punishment in their remit, or power to dismiss anybody.

One day I was teaching the admission procedure to a relatively junior nurse on her ward. Going through the admission procedure involved some paperwork and special forms used. These forms were indeed legal documents, and could in the event of a problem be used in a court case if necessary. They therefore had to be accurate and on completion signed by the nurse doing the admission of the patient. Included in the details were comments on those valuables which a patient brought in with them. Anything that was considered very valuable, with the patient's permission, was advised to be handed to the staff for safe keeping. A receipt would then be issued and the property put in the hospital safe until his discharge.

The patient I was admitting with this young nurse was an elderly man with leg ulcers, and in his wallet he had ten, ten pound notes. I asked the nurse if she thought this would constitute a risk to have so much money and how much did she think would be enough to buy such things as toiletries and cigarettes. She thought five pounds would be enough, but as he did not have any change I said that ten pounds would do. It was 1991 so it would really be only just enough to keep him going for a week, and he could always ask for more. The patient agreed to this so we took the £90 and gave him a receipt for that amount.

The next day the nurse came to me in tears and told me she had been threatened with dismissal by the nursing officer in charge because the ten pound note the patient retained had vanished, and the patient was saying it had been stolen, and the nursing officer said she was responsible and if she didn't pay it back she would be dismissed!

So once again I went into battle with somebody who had no real awareness of his role, evidenced by the way he appeared to have no awareness of the consequences of threatening an employee of the hospital without any evidence to support his allegations. I told him that that he had no authority to dismiss anybody. So after a rather heated session, he failed completely to understand that as it happened on his watch he was responsible. As he was so aware that he was right, I said, "Let's put it in writing and we will go together and see the hospital solicitor." That shut him up, but I had a real enemy now!

The ten pound note was found later in the day in the pyjama pocket of the coat the patient gave to his wife to take home for laundering! However no apology was forthcoming. I didn't expect one, but it showed me that he was a typical example of a man promoted to the level of his incompetence. He was a man well regarded by the then-administration as being a good manager, but coming from a service background myself, I reckoned that he would not have had the ability to achieve the rank of a junior N.C.O in the forces, and if he had, would not have held onto it for long.

As one of the goodies I had by working in all my spare time in the practice, I had eventually got the top-of-the-range car I had promised Pam all those years ago. It was a cracker and one morning I was showing a colleague of mine the works under the bonnet, when George, the aforementioned nursing officer, came out of the school. He came over to me and said sarcastically, "Well, well, what have we here, another new car?"

This rather annoyed me! "Hello George, did you see that programme on Channel Four on geriatric care last night?" I asked him.

"Indeed I did," he replied, "It was very good, did you not think so?"

"No," I said, "I was busy working at 9.00 p.m. whilst you were sitting on your bum watching TV, that's why I've got this, and you've only got a broken-down Toyota Sunny."

That really was the end of our relationship. He never spoke to me again!

I was now working only three days a week at the hospital, and it was beginning to get very difficult to cope with two roles, and I realised that I should make a decision about the future very soon or the pleasure that I was getting from both would soon sour; I would either make a major mistake in either role, or have to cut corners. I didn't want to do that, I wanted to give 100% to either of them, or one would have to go.

Times were changing, the clever people were taking over in the nursing profession and the emphasis seemed to be toward making the role of nurse into a manager of care rather than a carer of patients.

Also our esteemed director was moving on and a completely new generation of academics were going to be in charge, and many of my sidelines that had proved to be so useful to the staff – I was told – would no longer be the remit of the nursing school. I decided therefore the time had come to leave, go on holiday and make a final decision on return.

Pam and I had a very happy holiday in Scotland a few months before I retired from the NHS.

We spent the two weeks looking at the wildlife, had a fascinating trip on the Loch Ness, the boat being fitted with an echo sounder, and hoped to find the monster in the depths; it was a fruitless search, as so many others have found, but an enjoyable experience. Scotland really is a foreign country. I think the fact that it is so different is its attraction, even though we nearly froze to death at the top of the next mountain next to Ben Nevis!

On our return home we were rapidly forced to forget all about holidays when we got in the front door and found that the sun lounge and the consulting room adjoining the house were no longer adjoining, but had separated by some two inches due to subsidence. It was inspected by the insurance company, surveyors and builders were all called in and I was told that repairs were going to take some three months to jack it up and put it right. Fortunately the house was unaffected; we would not have to move out, but I would have to find another consulting room for the duration of the repair.

Helping the Lost!

I was fortunate in that a friend of mine, who had a osteopathic practice in the town, had a spare room, so I moved in there. It was very inconvenient as it was some distance away in the middle of the city, and also upstairs, and many of my patients had problems which did not permit them to climb stairs, so although the insurers paid the rent for it, I still suffered a considerable loss of earnings. It was however as happy a time as was possible; John and his two receptionists were good fun but busy people, so I could not force myself on them for too long in my quiet moments.

Work on my practice was completed to the day as promised, and I moved back in to an almost new set of rooms having had a lot of improvements made at the same time as the rebuild.

In retrospect however I think it was poor Pam who had to put up with all the mess. They dug out thirty-eight tons of clay under the rooms and filled the space with concrete, in the end it cost the insurer £29,000.

One day during the work, Pam heard a stentorian ring of the bell. When she opened the door, there stood a local councilor looking all superior. She knew who he was, but he did not have the manners to introduce himself. "What's all this noise?" he demanded. "It's getting on my wife's nerves." They lived a few doors away.

"Not half as much as on mine," she retorted. "Come with me," she said, took him round the back and showed him the hole. "Your council inspectors approved this building," she said, "twelve years ago, and this is the result and it's getting on my nerves too." He didn't know what to say and left in a hurry!

Do these stuffed shirts ever think of the image they convey, so different to the smarmy doorstep approach when they want your vote? We did not vote for him thereafter!

So I was back in business! My decision had of course been deferred about leaving the NHS by all this, but I finally made my mind up and tendered my resignation to go on my sixtieth birthday, which is what I did, and became self-employed for the first time in my life.

13

GETTING TO GRIPS WITH ROUTINE

I was finishing my role in the NHS, and the practice was paying its way after years in the red. The bank informed me that I was well and truly in the black, a great cause for celebration indeed!

I was very flattered when the school arranged a massive farewell party for me on the lunchtime of my sixtieth birthday. My family and most of my colleagues and a number of the administration attended, and even a couple of my own patients who had helped me at times with some of my hospital projects came along to join in the fun. I was showered with farewell gifts, including a model Rolls Royce; they wanted to get me a real one but the funds ran out, so I would have to put up with a Corgi one instead they said! I still have it on my desk as I write, and it reminds me of a very bittersweet day, but I had done my bit and with all the changes in the pipe line, it was time for me to move on again and concentrate properly on my practice.

I awoke the next morning to my new life, or at least the new chapter of my life, to find a whole raft of things to do both in the consulting room and the home, things that needed doing, but I had had little time to do them.

The garden needed attention, the car needed a good spring clean, the shed needed a new roof and so on. I gave myself a week to do all these things and to arrange a proper holiday for Pam and I, my daughter and granddaughter. I felt we all needed to let our hair down, and planned a fortnight in Malta. We'd all been many years before when I was in the RAF, and thought it would be great fun to revisit old haunts again in November.

My planned working week was now Monday to Friday with two mornings off to do such things as administration, banking, shopping and so on. Even in a small one-man band, there is a lot of paperwork to keep up with. I was still attending the college in London to give the occasional lecture, and the hospital under the new management asked me to talk to the nurses about alternative medicine; that was a surprise, but they were slowly waking up to its possibilities! My new life was therefore a lot more restful, and I found I no longer went to sleep in the bath at night when exhausted!

I now had time also to evaluate what I was doing and look for flaws in my thinking, and also had more chances to read the professional literature, instead of just scanning through it in a hurry and often missing some pearl of wisdom! So after all that, my retirement was busy but not overcrowded as my life had been with two different roles, but I was working from home and had the company of my wife, and the ability to nip indoors for a cup of coffee when I wanted one!

It was soon common knowledge that I was now a full-time practitioner, and along with more enquiries for treatment came various groups who wanted to know about acupuncture. I was never sure if they wanted information or entertainment, so produced two talks, and used the most appropriate one when I got to the venue of the talk, according to the mood of the meeting. Old ladies at a WI meeting needed a different approach to the business men at a Rotary club, and indeed medical groups needed a lot of preparation to get the message across as they really needed the facts spelled out professionally.

One Methodist church group had as their leader the wife of an orthopaedic consultant. Before I began she said to me, quite rudely I felt, that the group didn't want to hear any criticism of the NHS. I told her that my remit was to tell them about acupuncture, and as the invited speaker I would say what I wanted, and they could take what they wanted from my talk or not, and what did I want to talk about the NHS for anyway? However they listened in silence, and I think, taking their cue from their chairwoman, asked no questions! I don't think they dared!

Another group was the ME association; nobody turned up, to the disquiet of their chairman, who was a nice chap. I laughed and asked him what he expected of the membership, as a major symptom of ME is fatigue and probably all the members were too knackered to attend! He didn't quite see that point, he'd not got ME, so perhaps he didn't understand.

When a group of local GPs asked me to talk about medical acupuncture, before I started, having a coffee with them, one asked me what I did before I practiced acupuncture, and when I told them my history they accepted me at once. I was asked to talk to them for half an hour and they kept me there for nearly two hours! It was interesting to talk to people with open and enquiring minds, the senior one, after my explanation of terminology asked me, "If you don't use your belief system, doesn't it work?" I replied that I was not sure that I did believe all the words, but such terms as yin and yang, hot and cold, internal and external and so on meant different things in Chinese medicine to normal English usage, and were my model for practice, as he used antibiotics for infection, antihypertensive for high blood pressure and anti-inflammatory for inflammation, which terms would be indecipherable to a Chinese man, who would recognise those symptoms as they did, but use a different term to describe them.

So this meeting ended with a lot of goodwill generated, and one member went on eventually to study and practice acupuncture, so it was not a waste of time, I thought.

Other talks were a disaster. A young farmers' group asked me to talk and did their best from the word go to criticise and argue. I informed them I was not there to defend my therapy but to inform, and if they didn't have the manners to listen I would go, and promptly did, sent them a bill for petrol money, which they never paid; so I became wary of any group who asked me to talk, and thereafter I laid down conditions, which they either accepted, or I didn't go. The medical school at Addenbrookes still owe me my travelling expenses, but that was par for the course, I soon learned!

I got fed up with it quickly, often talking to closed minds, and getting busy with more and more people wanting help, I concentrated on my practice.

Advertising was much the same; the local press would phone me and ask my opinion on something that had been reported nationally when some celebrity had been treated for something drastic by acupuncture, picked my brains, and then offered me a discount on an ad in their paper, which had a circulation of 60,000 souls I was told!

So I soon came to recognise that personal recommendation was the best form of advertising, and judging by the number of patients I was getting, this was the way to go. After all most of my patients were 'refugees from general medicine' and my approach was preferable for them, but contained in my treatment was an element of teaching; the majority of citizens of this land know little about their bodies, or such concepts as disease, or either how health is maintained by the body, and what really happens when it all goes horribly wrong! The usual statement is, 'I've caught a disease'.

My basic premise was that of Hahneman, the father of homeopathy, 'There is no such thing as disease, only diseased individuals'.

When asked what I meant, I would reply, 'Have you ever seen a lump of disease?' to which of course the answer is no. Rather a simplistic statement but some understood it.

Disease is the experience of the individual when the body's immune system for example is overwhelmed by a virus or a bacterium, it gets into the body, via the mouth, or skin or whatever route, and the body cannot destroy it, then the body reacts in a specific way: for example if the bug is of say tuberculosis, you will then experience a well-charted pattern known for years as TB, if it is a pneumococcus your body will respond by a swelling and consolidation of part of the lung, and that is known as pneumonia. That is what is commonly called a disease! Also if the rhino virus enters your nostril and your immune system cannot overcome it, you will respond with a runny nose, and that we refer to as a cold! It's not the bacterium, it's the bodily response to it that is the disease. However the choice is yours how you respond; some people get a cold and are dead on their feet, others say 'I haven't got time to be poorly' and get on with their lives, others use it as a means of avoiding work and so on. We all react to disease due to the way we think, our moral code, our age, fortitude or impatience, the rich pattern of reactions to disease in other words; we make a choice and may not realise we have done so. And sometimes the invading principle is so overwhelming, we succumb and possibly die.

Also, you can be ill and not diseased, and you can be diseased and not ill, so all these permutations have to be thought about by the practitioner. I always tell new practitioners, when they come into your office try and establish if the patient is ill or just not well, in other words not fitting into the world around him!

So when the clever sceptics try and trip me up with the usual, 'Can you cure bronchitis', for example, I reply, 'No, you've not been listening, but I can treat the person who has it'. And that is what the practice of acupuncture is all about! Trying to modify the patient's response, not kill the cause, even if you do know the cause.

One day a young married woman with two young children asked to see me. She was rather scruffily dressed and had a rather haunted look about her. She said she was not sleeping well, but did not want to sleep too deeply because when she did she had nightmares about her children being killed or abducted. Her own GP had seen her, done all the usual blood tests and could find no reason for her problem, so offered her either Valium, 'the panacea for all ills', or to be referred to the pyschiatrist as he thought she was depressed. I started my questionnaire as usual and found that she had been like this for some six months. She was a translator of technical journals for a major publishing house; she'd already made a couple of mistakes, and was worried that she would be sacked. I asked her about her home, she said it was a lovely house but she had never felt comfortable there. Her husband was a teacher at a public school in the Midlands and he commuted daily.

She was a graduate from a good Scottish university, where she had met her husband some five years ago. They were both on the same teaching course, and on graduating went to work at the same school together in the south of Scotland. I asked her why then did they come down south to work, she said rather shame-facedly that her husband had big ideas and felt the only way he could progress in teaching, to get to the top, was in the private sector.

"It sounds as though you didn't agree with that decision," I said.

"No," she said, "not really I didn't, but wanted him to get on."

"Why didn't you agree?" I asked. She said that she was older than him, and he came from an upper-class family and she felt he got to the university almost as a rite of passage, but she was from a working-class family and had to struggle to get there.

"Do you get on with his friends?" I asked.

"No, I don't understand them, they're very shallow people I think," she replied.

"When were you last happy?" I asked.

"When we were together at our first school." She named the school, it so happened that I knew the area having spent a holiday there in the caravan only the previous year.

Getting to Grips with Routine

"The one down by the river," I asked her, her face lit up.

"Oh yes," she said, "you know it, oh it was a lovely school!"

"So, you have few friends then," I observed.

"No, not locally," she replied. "It gets a bit lonely at times with only two young children who are at school all day."

I thought for a moment, whatever I said next was going to make or break this situation.

Treatment with needles is one thing, but she was fearful for her life and family; after all, what she was doing was reacting to the situation she found herself in. I couldn't change that, drugs would only have taken the raw edges away temporarily, then she'd have gone back to square one, and acupuncture may have modified her feelings for a while with the same result. This was different!

About a month before I had bought a book by a well-known writer on social affairs. He had conducted interviews in his home area where she had first worked with her husband. It recounted interviews with some thirty of the locals.

It was a very depressed area with little work for anyone, and in fact had been like this for years. The book dealt with local people from the young to the elderly, from those who could remember hiring themselves at the fair each year to the farmers or big houses, to present day youths on benefits who had to survive with all the despair that came with that sort of life. So it was a sort of microcosm of the area, and the author used the local dialects to tell his story.

I took it down off my shelf and asked her if she had read it, I told her what it was about and I said she could read it if she'd like to. She thanked me, and I then treated her insomnia and fear with acupuncture, and arranged another session the following week.

The following week she came back in looking a little less tired. She had had better nights and she only one or two nasty dreams, but less than before.

"Did you like the book?" I asked.

"Oh yes, isn't it wonderful, it's written just the way they speak up there," she said with a smile and handed it to me.

"You've not finished it surely?" I said.

"No, I've only read the first chapter, it's wonderful. It's just the way they speak."

"Well you finish it, and I'll see you next week," I said and treated her again using the same points.

When she came back a week later, she looked good, she was sleeping well she said, and no more dreams. I saw her five more times until she was completely symptom-free. On the last visit she came in with a big smile on her face.

"I feel good," she said.

"Good, have you finished the book?" I asked her.

She went a bit red and put her hand into her bag and was still for a minute.

"Well let me have it," I said, holding out my hand.

Oh dear, she's lost it I thought, but then she took the book out, turned it over in her hands looking at it, and said quietly and somewhat ruefully, "It wasn't very good up there was it?"

"No," I said, "you've been living in the past, it's today that matters, coping with that."

I think it's the old story, those to whom she had turned for help heard what she said, but didn't listen, and in particular didn't listen to what she didn't say!

Again and again I found this to be the problem, judgements made and given taking the easiest way out, and in those days, it was usually a packet of Valium!

One day a tall, suave, well-dressed and well-spoken young man came to see me for treatment for persistent frontal headaches. Before he sat down he told me that he was a practicing homosexual.

"What's that got to do with me?" I asked.

He replied that his GP said that that was the cause of his headaches!

"Sorry," I said, " I can't see the connection."

He replied that his GP said he therefore had a stressful lifestyle.

"Do you"? I asked.

"We all do in these recessionary times, I'm in business but we get by," he said.

"Who is we?" I asked.

"My partner is also my business partner, we run a small holding together," he replied, "and we've been together for fifteen years and never had a cross word, and the business gives us a good living."

"How long have you had the headaches?" I asked him.

"Eight years," he said, "usually over the eyes and very annoying."

"What investigation has been done?" I asked.

"I've had none," he said.

"What treatment have you had then?" I said.

"None apart from a packet of codeines every two months," he replied.

"Have you ever been examined or had any other investigations?" I asked.

"Not in any detail," he replied.

I have learned over the years to always take a persistent headache seriously. I physically examined him and found little of note, particularly neurologically, but the position of the pain in his head I felt was relevant. But on detailed examination I found that he had an old appendix operation scar, and when I prodded it firmly he cried out in pain. I then found that his kidney on the same side was palpable, sore and enlarged.

"Do you get up at night to have a pee?" I asked.

"Yes," he said, "usually about four times. It's very disturbing, but I'm used to it now."

In Chinese medicine the kidney meridian ends above the eyes, hence the headache, so I then got him to pass a urine specimen. It was coloured like mud and had blood in it.

"So when did your headaches start?" I asked again.

"Eight years ago," he said.

"And when did you have your appendix out?" I persisted.

He frowned, "Eight years ago, now I come to think of it."

"You've got a drainage problem," I told him. "Your ureter, the tube that runs from your kidney to your bladder, is probably kinked by adhesions from that operation, so the urine stagnates in the kidney. As it can't get out quickly it gets infected."

I gave him a letter to take to his GP and told him to insist that he examined him. But the GP was not amused and told him to keep away from these people like me! "They don't know what they're doing," he said, but he did examine him this time. I had briefed the patient! He took some bloods, on return of which with the results he sent him for kidney radiograph, and when the X rays were seen, sent him to the urologist who confirmed my findings, and then congratulated me on my diagnosis!

The patient was treated surgically and with antibiotics and the headaches went, never to return, at least not for that reason! This poor man had suffered eight years of pain due to the prejudice of his GP, a salutary lesson to all to keep their feelings to themselves.

A young nurse phoned me one evening from the hospital and came to see me the same evening.

She was in a dilemma; how could she hurt people who were already ill by sticking needles in them and causing them more distress? This of course, if she could not find an answer to the problem, would mean that she would have to leave the profession which she loved; she was a senior student and would be taking her final exams within the next six months. She came to see me at 8.30 p.m., tired from a day on duty. She looked tired. I had met her before, two years before I retired. She had married an RAF man who was based in Yorkshire, and not wanting to leave nursing, had transferred her training to a local hospital in the north, but to my surprise, here she was again back with her original course.

"How can I help?" I asked.

She outlined her problem with tears in her eyes as she spoke and conveyed to me a sense of her own unworthiness in that she could not help the sick if she had to hurt them sometimes.

"Tell me about yourself," I said, "not your immediate problem."

She'd had a happy childhood, brought up in a service family, and had lived abroad a lot. Her father was a senior army officer, mother a teacher of classics; it was with her siblings a very happy loving family life, only disturbed by all the different postings, but stable in the circumstances.

She came to this hospital after her A levels to fulfill her ambition to be a nurse, but after nine months fell in love with a very handsome airman, who she said was destined for higher things. He was waiting to go to OCTU for officer training.

They were married from her parent's house in the stockbroker belt, and left for an idyllic honeymoon in Mauritius. The hospital had been sorry to see her leave, and allowed her to transfer to the local hospital near her husband's unit. She had been happy at the new location, but things went badly wrong with the marriage. Her husband turned out to be an alcoholic, and when drunk beat her up. This went on for a few months until she decided to report him to the RAF authorities. She saw the families officer, the padre, and even after a lot of trouble the unit C.O but nobody believed that this well regarded young man could be like that, the M.O offered her Valium as usual, but she had had enough and started planning to leave him.

It was at the time of IRA terrorist attacks, and the unit was under strict security, there was a lot of coming and going, the men being posted in and out, but her husband did not go being in a key post.

One night in sheer desperation she packed her bag, crawled out under the wire onto the main road, thumbed a lift and went to her parents house in Warwickshire. She had not told them of her problems, but when she got home to her distress found it was closed up with a for sale board outside. The neighbours told her that her parents had separated, the house was up for sale, and her father had left the service and was working at a public school in Scotland. She managed to trace him on the telephone; he couldn't take her in, he only had a one bedroom school flat, nor did he know where his wife was. He advised her to go back to Peterborough and finish her course there, it would at least give her a roof over her head and then he would help her financially regarding the divorce she wanted.

So she came back to the fold and continued her course, she was welcomed back by her friends, but she was a very different young lady to the one she had been when she was single.

"And that's it," she said, her eyes full of pain. "What do I do?"

It was now 12.30 a.m. and I was feeling pretty drained. What it must have cost her to unload that lot I don't know, but for a sensitive and well-brought-up girl, I could sense that she was absolutely appalled at what had happened, that only happened in books! She obviously felt a sense of guilt, thinking it was her fault, but such is life. Her reaction to all this, the worry, the unworthiness, the sleepless nights, the beating up, and now the injection failure was too much.

We sat in silence for a little while, I held her hand while we talked it through, and then put her on my couch and treated her for sadness, and comforted her with a foot massage. She dozed off for a few minutes, I then woke her up, fetched her a cup of tea, then put her in the car and took her back to the nurses' home.

Two days later she sent me a little note: 'Thank you for your help, can you treat me for an aching face, I can't stop smiling at people!'

No, you can't always change the cause of the patient's problem, but you can change the way they respond to it, and that is always my main thrust of attack. However, sometimes the problem is caused by the patient's unwillingness to take responsibility for their actions.

An eighteen-year-old youth came to see me on the insistence of his mother who was distressed to see her son's rheumatoid arthritis deteriorate to the point where he could hardly walk. He was dragged along very reluctantly to the appointment by his father.

He'd had to give up all sports and was now working only three days a week in a shop but was now finding it very difficult to do even that because of his swollen knees and ankle joints. He had been treated, according to his father, with anti-rheumatic drugs for three years, but rarely took them and failed to keep his appointment with the rheumatologist. He therefore had little chance of getting anywhere so far as his health was concerned.

This rather aggressive and arrogant young man plonked himself down in front of me with the attitude, go on do what you want, this is all a waste of time!

After taking as full a history as I could, which was difficult because of his reluctance to answer even simple questions, I examined his very swollen hot painful joints and his spindly wasted legs.

"Why don't you take your tablets?" I asked him.

"Waste of time," he replied in a very surly voice.

"Well, that doesn't help," I remarked.

"That's right," said his father, "you tell him, he won't talk to us."

"No, please," I said, "let me handle this."

It was obvious I had to get through to him, and shouting at him was not the way to get any cooperation. He'd got to be shamed into a realisation of what he was doing to his body, and I would have to take a tortuous path into his mind!

"You're eighteen," I said, "have you got a girlfriend?"

"Why?" he answered belligerently.

"Well have you?" I went on.

"What's that got to do with it?" he asked.

I ignored that reply, "Do you love her?"

"Suppose so," he said reluctantly,

"And do you plan to ask her to marry you?" I asked him.

"Maybe," he replied.

"And have kids?" I asked him.

"Yes, what's all this got to do with it then?" he muttered.

"You've got a nerve," I observed.

"What d'you mean?" he said startled.

I pulled my chair closer to him and looked him straight in the eye, "You'd force yourself on a woman, get her pregnant and then the resulting child will end up with a father in a wheelchair, and a wife with a husband who can't do anything only moan about pain in his legs that don't work anyway? Do you think she's going to like being married to a cripple, pushing you around? Big deal eh?"

He looked nonplussed at that.

His father chipped in, "That's right, you tell him."

"No please, leave it to me," I said. "What do you eat?" I asked him. "You mother and your GP would have told you about dietary needs."

"Steak and chips," he replied.

"Oh come on, at breakfast, lunch and dinner?" I asked him.

"That's right."

"What do you drink?" I asked him.

"Coke, about twelve bottles a day," he replied sullenly.

"Is that your daily food intake?" I asked incredulously.

"Yes, that's it," he replied.

"Do you want to get better?" I said.

By now some of the arrogance had gone, and he was looking quite woebegone!

"Course I do," he muttered.

"You're not going to do it your way," I said. "I'll treat you but you must do as I say for a fortnight, and if you are not 50% better within two weeks I'll give you your money back, or at least your father's money! OK?"

"What do I do then?" he asked.

"Eat nothing but boiled fish, chicken and rice, and drink only spring water, and come and see me next week, oh and yes, take your tablets."

I treated him with the appropriate acupuncture regime and saw him a week later: he could then walk! After the second treatment he continued to progress and by the end of the month he was playing football, and was working full time again, and virtually pain-free!

Most of my work was with those I refer to as refugees from conventional medicine, those who had little or no success with their conventional treatment, or felt that the success was limited in that their disease had been treated, but they had been left out of the equation.

Children by and large are unable to make such fine distinctions, and although I saw few children, one has hopefully the ability to make an impact on their young lives that helps, not only them but their family.

A little lass called June, who was about seventeen years old but had a mental age of ten, was the much loved daughter of her widowed mother. They lived in the Midlands and had to come to see me by train, which June really enjoyed! She had no close relatives to help out with what could be a very difficult situation, and relied upon only a few friends, but when the going got tough, as is so common, they coped alone. Her husband, a solicitor, had died of cancer some three years previously. June missed him terribly, and had developed rheumatoid arthritis after her father's death, which affected her hands and wrists, which was a major problem to them both, as they were into country sports and both loved horse riding.

She was a sweet child and quite biddable, but in all cases like this I always wondered what would happen to the child when her parent died. Her mother was quite open about this and was prepared to discuss it, but it did distress her, and as she said, we take it a day at a time and can't think too far ahead. We enjoy each day as it comes. June was of course very attached to her mother and drew strength from her. I treated her successfully for the pain in her hands, seeing her once a week for a month. One day when they came into the office, June asked if she could go to the toilet first.

When she had left the room her mother said to me that she was glad to talk to me on her own. "We've got a major problem now," she said, "June wants a baby! What am I going to do? The people I've spoken to have been little help."

"Do you want me to talk to her?" I asked.

"Do you think you can dissuade her?" she said hopefully.

June came back into the room, she sat down and I went through all the usual routine and treatments.

I looked up at her, "June, you've got something worrying you," I said, "what's up?"

"I want a baby," she said, and sniffed the tears back.

"Do you really?" I replied. "That's lovely, do you know any?"

She told me that the young couple who lived next door had just had a little girl and she'd been allowed to cuddle it and couldn't stop talking about it from morning to night.

"You love babies then, and now want one of your own. We all have something we want. Do you know what I want? In fact in the same way as you nearly burst wanting a baby, so do I for what I want."

"What's that?" she asked tremulously.

"Well I want a Jaguar car, six-cylinder, post-office red with cream leather seats, a nice radio fitted, special tyres and all the other fittings you can get nowadays."

"Do you?" she said. "Why don't you get one then?"

I gave a mock sigh. "Ah, well that's the problem," I replied, "those cars are so special, just like a baby, they need constant attention to keep them on the road, cost an awful lot of money, and because of that you don't have a lot of time or money for anything else. They are so expensive."

June looked down at her hands, "Yes, I suppose so," she said tearfully and went home with her mother.

I saw them again the following week. Her mother said she'd not mentioned a baby again, so I must have said the right thing!

This is a problem with healthy young mentally handicapped children. Do you let them follow their natural instincts or not? They have the same instincts as the rest of us, but when the carers die, what then?

Another category of patient who came to see me was those who had been treated for their presenting condition, but did not progress because they either interfered, sometimes unwittingly, with their treatment, or would not take medicines as prescribed.

A fifty-year-old lady came in one day with a very irritating skin disease. It was so severe she had scratched herself, and had many unsightly lesions on her head and limbs, and wore a long dress with long sleeves and also a scarf on her head to hide this hideous scarring. She told me that she had been given creams for it, but it did not help and she thought they were making it worse. She had been given a diagnosis, but from experience I felt it was wrong and that this was a drug rash, but she said she was on no drugs. The trouble with that statement is that many people think drugs mean addictive substances such as heroin or cocaine!

As I questioned her on her lifestyle and medical history, I discovered that she was a retired financial adviser at a national bank, but had left the bank to help her husband in business. She enjoyed the work, and also being with her husband all day was to her very pleasant!

He was a thermal engineer and had started his own firm near Leicester making industrial ovens, and she spent a lot of her time with him testing and developing these pieces of equipment. It was rather hot work, and as it was now summer, the heat in the workshop was sometimes unbearable. But it was lucrative and the orders kept coming in, even from China, she said proudly, and they wanted to visit that country to go to a trade fair the next year.

It was obvious she had a fulfilling life and worked very hard, but she looked tired. She said she was a poor sleeper.

"Does the rash worry you at night in bed? It must be very difficult to sleep, does it keep you awake?" I asked her.

"No, that doesn't," she said. She emphasised the 'that'.

"Oh well, what does?" I asked.

"It's the cramps in my legs, they often keep me awake, I had to see my GP about it and she gave me some tablets," she replied.

"Do they help?" I asked.

"Oh yes," she said, "they do help a lot."

"What are they?" I asked, "are they Quinine, that's the standard one for cramps?"

"That's the one," she said, "a little white one."

By now alarm bells were ringing in my head!

"Let's get back to the job you do," I said. "You say it gets very hot in the workshop, do you sweat a lot?"

"Gallons," she replied.

"Do you take plenty of salt to replace what you've sweat?"

"No I never take any salt, it's bad for you I'm told," she replied.

"Not even added to cooking?" I asked her.

"No none, never touch it."

"And do you replace the fluid you sweat?"

"Oh yes I drink gallons, get very thirsty, why?" she asked.

"One more thing: what do you replace the fluid with, what do you drink?"

"I drink tonic water, lovely stuff! Something wrong with that?" she asked, noting my grimace! Now I had the answer to her problem!

"Your cramps are a classic sign of reduced blood sodium levels, that is salt. You sweat, you say, and so lose a lot of salt from your blood, that is the cause of your cramps. Quinine eases the cramp, but tonic water is full of Quinine, and with your tablets added, you have got Quinine poisoning from a huge intake of the drug and tonic water, hence your drug rash," I told her.

She looked shattered. "Did you tell your GP about the tonic water and your aversion to salt?" I asked.

"No, I didn't think it had anything to do with my problems," she replied in astonishment.

Not on any drugs indeed! By stopping the Quinine, adding a small amount of salt to her diet, and drinking water instead of tonic, in two weeks both her cramps and the skin rash disappeared!

There are many stories told about acupuncture and the marvellous benefits it can give, and those who criticise it know less than nothing about it, told usually by those who have a particular agenda or are ignorant of reality, and just don't know what life is all about.

One of these is the question I am often asked: can acupuncture stop people smoking?

I don't think it can, but if the person will stop, it will help him remain a non-smoker. Smoking is a bad habit which has progressed into an addiction, and that's the problem. It's got stuck, as it were, in the system, and the body gets used to it, misses its presence, and reacts by saying 'What are you doing? if you don't have a fag, I'll make you feel awful,' so the fag eases the feelings of disquiet!

It's therefore a social as well as a personal problem. But to treat somebody with addiction, there needs to be an understanding on the part of the patient of what has happened to him, and the need to want to give up, and the realisation of just what nicotine is doing to his physiology. After all, nobody made him smoke in the first place. It was a choice he'd made, and not a good one!

One day a young woman phoned me and asked to see me because she wanted to give up her twenty-a-day habit.

"Why?" I asked.

"I'm an athlete," she said, "and it's ruining my wind," she replied.

"Are you a good athlete?" I asked her.

"Yes," she said. "I'm county standard."

"Jolly good," I said, "would you in time like to become an Olympic champion?"

"Oh yes," she enthused, "that's what I want more than anything."

"Well give up smoking, then," I replied. "You've got the best reason in the world to do it, and think of the pleasure you'd get if you gave up and won a gold. You don't need me!"

"Is that all you've got to say?" she snarled.

"Yes," I said. "Good day," and put the phone down.

She wanted somebody to blame for her failure, and it wasn't going to be me! That may sound harsh, but she was the author of her own misfortune, and was not going to succeed in a sport that required total commitment and discipline required unless she gave up the habit and exercised a bit of personal discipline! Like so many others she'd got her priorities wrong.

There are stories of those who are over ninety and smoke like chimneys, the 'It's not done me any harm' brigade, which proves my previous point that it's the reaction to the problem that is the problem, rather than the problem itself.

One day a sixty-three-year-old man came to see me with a cold, pulseless left leg, with which he suffered severe cramp at night stopping him sleeping.

"And don't tell me to stop smoking because I'm not going to," he stated even before he sat down.

"I didn't ask you about that, but I would have got round to it, believe me," I said.

"How many do you smoke?" I asked.

"Sixty a day," he replied.

"But that's one every ten minutes, or ten hours' smoking a day!" I said in amazement.

"That's right," he said, "I light up a fresh one as I finish the other."

"Have you taken advice," I asked him, "about your leg?"

"Yes, and all they want to do is to do some sort of bypass, and I'm not having that, and they said they wouldn't do it anyway unless I stop smoking, so blow them, they're not going to tell me what to do!"

This was quite a challenge, but I agreed to see what I could do over four weeks, promising him nothing. So I treated his leg with acupuncture and massage after I had assured myself that he had no thrombosis, and at the end of the four weeks his leg was functioning normally, the pulse was back, but he was still smoking like a chimney!

It was now crunch time and what I did next would be critical. "How long do you live in your family?" I asked.

"Oh, most of us live to about eighty-five," he said. "Why?"

"Well," I said looking straight in the eye. "You've got another twenty-five years or so of your life left, but at the end of it you're going to die." He looked startled.

"So?" he said.

"Well you're going to have a dreadful death if you don't stop smoking."

His face went white, he stood up, threw down my fee, walked out and slammed the door behind him. I never saw him again. Oh these smokers!

14

DAY TO DAY PROBLEMS

As I became known by reputation the patients came from far and wide to see me. I needed more time to rest, and we used the caravan for more holidays than most people have!

On one of our many forays into the north, we visited one of the many famous ruined abbeys, and one afternoon found what we thought was the most beautiful one of all, Reivaux Abbey.

We wandered, delighting in the utter peace and tranquility and beauty of the ruin. It was warm, the sun shone, the sheep feeding on the lush grass of the site were munching away – the only sound in the silence of that lovely afternoon. Pam and I got separated; she wandered into what was left of the nave, and I was left leaning on a low wall in the cloister reveling in the peace and quiet. Before me, the sheep fed. They are such quiet animals and appear to threaten nobody.

Suddenly two low-flying Lightning jets from the nearest airfield appeared, flying straight at us in the abbey, and as they came over the top, turned up to the sky with afterburners burning. The noise was appalling for a few moments, and then back to utter silence again! The sheep carried on munching, it was still warm, the sun still shone. Suddenly a man stood beside me – I hadn't noticed him before, being engrossed in the scene – a tall man in a Sherlock Holmes outfit with a deerstalker hat, and without looking at me he said, "If you and I, sir, were two monks 800 years ago, standing here, and heard that cacophony, we would have gone rushing in to the abbot. 'Father Abbot' we'd have cried, 'we've just seen the devil himself come hurtling out of the sky spitting flames and roaring threats, what shall we do?' And for our pains," he continued, "we would have been put on bread and water for a month, and not allowed to leave our cells." He turned to me and smiled, "You see, only the abbot was allowed to see the devil!" he raised his hat and said, "Good day to you," and walked away!

I have no idea who he was, but by his remarks he made a very bright day even brighter!

Meanwhile the animals continued to graze peacefully, not in the least discomforted by our presence or the commotion, which I feel says something about the attitude and psychology of sheep to the presence of the devil!

I was now quite adept at towing a caravan, and we found a lot of pleasure in using it. The problem was collecting it from storage the night before we used it, filling it up with all the goodies necessary for civilised living, and at the end of the break having to reverse the process before we took it back to store. We found it unwise to leave anything of value in it. We'd already had a lot of our possessions stolen on one occasion just before a holiday; insurance covered the cost, but did not cover the distress we felt finding that some yob had desecrated our property.

We therefore decided to sell the van and buy a mobile home which we did not need to restock each time we wanted to use it, so we purchased a very nice thirty-five foot static van on a secure seaside site, and found we could then go to it, being only an hour or so away when we had a break of only a day if necessary, and it became a useful amenity for the rest of the family when they wanted a break, or to come with us, as it had two good bedrooms.

We visited Malta again just after our purchase; we'd been the previous year, after I retired from the NHS. We rented an up-market villa in one of the villages and took again with us our daughter Gillian and our granddaughter Rebecca for a two week break.

The holiday was a disaster. A few days prior to the holiday Rebecca was unwell with a mild tummy ache. I advised Gillian to get the GP to see her. He thought she had a simple tummy upset, but the ache persisted, and the day before the holiday she called in the GP again. A different one arrived this time, and thought she was just exited at the prospect of the holiday, and gave his approval to carry on.

After a good flight, we settled into our five-star villa, but the next day Rebecca was very sluggish, so we rested, but that evening when she had gone to bed, I went in to say goodnight and could sense something was wrong. I felt her abdomen and it was as tight as a drum, she had a temperature and a nasty smelling breath. She had all the signs of acute appendicitis.

I found a GP on call and told him the problem. He was with us from the other side of the island in fifteen minutes – he must have broken every speed limit – took one look at her, told me to get her into the car and follow him as quickly as possible to the main hospital in Valetta where she was operated on within the hour. A huge 'appendix mass' was found and removed, she was filled up with antibiotics and she survived. It was all a bit dodgy but poor Rebecca had a very painful holiday!

The ward staff were first-class. Both the ward sisters were trained at Great Ormond Street, the leading London paediatric teaching hospital. They were kindness itself, and naturally very good nurses. It was the practice in Malta for mothers to stay with their child during illness, an excellent idea I felt, and so we had to find a bed for Gillian, and feed her, and relieve her every couple of days so she could get a bath and a good meal. Poor Gillian, she went through a lot that fortnight. Sickness in a foreign country with a different culture is most upsetting for one's self, but to have a dearly-loved child seriously ill is dreadful. All in all, a lot of effort for a couple of thousand pounds, but Rebecca did well, the ward staff called her their 'little English angel' and spoilt her as much as they could. I found out a lot about the health service in Malta that fortnight. They were very badly-paid, and the day before we left, having spent most of our time at hospital we had spent little and had a large amount of spending money left. Pam suggested we give it to the staff to do what they wanted with it, preferably go out and have a good time and enjoy themselves, which we were told the next time we visited the island that they had done so.

So it was with great relief that we arrived back home to pick up the pieces. We planned to return the following year; we'd all four of us had our appendixes removed now, so that would not happen again!

I was often asked as a practitioner for advice on not only matters medical but on such diverse subjects as tax, house insurance, car maintenance, matrimonial matters and so on. My response, of course, varied on the amount of knowledge I had on any subject. If I did not have that degree of expertise, I would say 'I don't know, but I know a man who does' and as in medicine refer the questioner to an expert, and after all these years in practice, I did know quite a few!

Sometimes people would ask for advice on serious health matters which they had been unable to find an answer to – no Wikipedia in those early days!

A woman asked me one day if I could help her seventeen-year-old son, who was a bed wetter. This is an unusual problem in a young man, and there are a variety of causes for a boy of that age to suffer this problem, from simple anxiety right through to physical disease such as malignancy. So this was serious; she had not taken him to see a consultant urologist, she didn't know what that was, he had seen his GP who had "given him some tablets" but it didn't help.

I asked her about the boy; he was at a public school but not a boarder, a good sportsman and wanted to join the army, and she thought he should go to Sandhurst as his deceased father had in the past.

I had to advise her that he had no chance of joining the armed forces, as bed wetting in a society in which men lived close together was unacceptable, and suggested she get a consultant appointment as soon as possible. She was grateful for my help but ended by saying that she thought acupuncture could cure the problem!

I can recall one remarkable example of bed wetting when I was in charge of a ward whilst at an RAF hospital. A young man, a junior N.C.O, was admitted to my ward with the problem. We were near London and often had patients sent to us for final diagnosis and disposal. We were near the central medical establishment where the medical details of all serving men were kept, and decisions regarding their employment depending upon their state of health were made there. This young man stayed with us for a couple of days before his appointment. I was on night duty at the time, and each night about 3.00 a.m. he would come into the office and apologise, "Sorry chief, I've done it again", rather dolefully and full of apology. I'd give him clean sheets and he'd go back to sleep. I'd looked through his notes; he was in the service for twelve years and had completed five, he knew how serious this was and had been advised following masses of investigations that if they could find no answer to the problem, he would have to be discharged on medical grounds. He had apparently said to one investigator that he liked the service and wanted to get on well.

I went on nights off, and on my return, my first job was to process this young man, who had been discharged on medical grounds. I called him into the office and did the paper work and sent him to get his final pay, hand in his uniform and so on. I told him to report back to me on completion of this task. He came back in about half an hour. I invited him to sit down and have a cup of coffee, handed him his discharge papers and travel warrant and train times.

He still had a bit of a hang dog expression, but thanked me for "not getting on at him as everyone else had", he said. He finished his coffee, and I said, "Well, you're a civilian now."

"That's right," he said.

"Well," I said, "I can't do anything to you as you are not in the service anymore."

"That's right," he said.

"Will you answer me a question, honestly?" I asked him.

He thought for a moment, looked up at me and smiled.

"OK," he said.

"Was it all worth it?" I asked.

His face split into a huge grin. "Every bloody minute of it," he replied laughing. "I'm out!"

"Well I expected as much," I said, "but you've given a lot of people a lot of work and cost a lot of money, if you'd put that amount of energy into your job, you'd be an Air Vice Marshall by now. I'll give you ten out of ten for effort."

"But I never wanted to be an Air Vice Marshall," he replied. "Goodbye, I'll miss my train if I'm not careful, don't want to do that!"

He grinned and shook hands, went back to Cornwall and home. He'd have to live with his conscience after that, if he had one!

15

THE DOOR CLOSES BUT ANOTHER OPENS

Unnoticed by me, I was getting older although enjoying my work, but working five twelve-hour days was going to take a toll of my health, but like most people when feeling well, I thought I was indestructible.

We were now enjoying the benefits of a much higher income – and paying a lot of tax, business rates, professional fees and all that goes with running a business, however small – but one well-remembered day I was pulled up sharp. Out shopping, I felt a pain in my chest. It disappeared when I stopped, but I knew what it was; not enough to send me running for help but the warning was there, I was determined to get on with life if I could and slow down a bit! I obviously had a furred-up coronary artery.

My main reaction to this was disappointment that my body had let me down, but on reflection soon realised that it was I who had let it down! This occurred just before Christmas 1998, and in February I was going with my son to the Maldives, for a visit to once again enjoy the fun I'd had when as a young man in the RAF. I had spent a memorable posting to RAF Gan for a year in 1964, the RAF's far eastern airfield used as a refuelling point for air traffic between UK and our overseas possessions in that part of the globe.

Pam was not keen on me going, I had not told her about my chest pain or she would have vetoed it on the spot. Also to her, the name Gan was anathema. When I was posted there, she had to get out of married quarters and stay at her parents' home with the three children, and had a most unhappy time. However plans were finalised. I knew I had to be careful on the holiday, my son would be scuba diving, but I would spend my time reading, or cycling if possible.

We arrived at Gatwick on the Sunday evening, and waited some two hours for a slot to take off. We were routed down over Africa to Mombasa because Sadam Hussein was sabre rattling at that time, then on to the Maldives. This was a long drag, but I must admit even though no longer young, I enjoyed all of the twenty-two hours' flight, and arriving at Male, the capital, was taken to a noisy hotel in the middle of the town, and left next morning on a small aircraft for the journey to Gan, some 400 miles to the south.

I was lucky with my holiday reading, it was an old book by Mark Twain called *A Tramp Abroad*. I had read it many years before, the tale of the author's obligatory grand tour, written about 1856, and described his journey with a travelling companion. Each place he visited he found some amusing anecdote to tell, some hilarious and some sad, but with the expertise of a good writer, wrote a book that the reader found difficult to put down!

I had, as I said, read it before, when as kids during the war we used to go round the houses asking for unwanted items for the war effort, as it was known. We collected all kinds of rubbish, from pots and pans to be melted down to make Spitfires, we were told, and books which were 'comforts' for the troops. At the end of a day's collecting, we went through our acquisitions and naughtily removed items we found attractive to us. One of the books was this one, but when I left home to join the RAF it disappeared, and although I searched all second-hand bookshops, I never again found a copy, until one day a patient came to see me who was a librarian. She admired my collection of books above my desk and we got talking about favourite books. I mentioned this book, but although she had read some of Mark Twain she did not know this one. The following week she came for her follow up appointment and handed me a leather-bound rather scruffy volume and said, "Is this the one?"

It was indeed; she had been sent a tea chest of old books from the main library for disposal or to be shredded if not wanted, and there it was. I could have kissed her – I didn't, as I did not want to get arrested! But it was wonderful to get hold of it again.

So this entertained me on the holiday in which sadly I found that I could not do those things I did previously as a youngster; my heart would not let me, the flesh was weak although the spirit was more than willing, but I could read!

The journey down to Gan in a small aircraft was wonderful. Flying at some 5000 feet we could see all the other islands spread out before us – the Indian Ocean from on high is so beautiful – but as we came in to land, it was like coming home, the same palm trees, white beaches, sunshine, the native people looked just the same – I thought they were the same, but this was forty years on. Little appeared to have changed on the island; there was the same post office, the same Astra cinema still working, and still called the Astra! The same road up to the hotel, which was the old mess; the accommodation was changed and brought up to date with en-suite bathrooms, but all the views were the same. It really felt like home!

All the many trees which had been only bushes in my previous stay were now fully grown, lovely kanda trees, palms and a flowering bush like a hibiscus, all combined to give an impression of paradise!

The first evening just before dinner, my son Graham and I wandered up the traffic-free road to the causeway linking Gan to the next island in the atoll, called Fehdu, and looked across the water. When I was there before, the causeway was damaged, and Fehdu was inaccessible apart from by boat, or by wading through the warm water. It was also out-of-bounds to us personnel. It was absolutely quiet and tranquil, as we stood there drinking in the beauty of the place, the flying foxes, fruit bats like big black crows, flew over on their way to their roosts for the night, and a column of smoke arose from some cooking fire above the palms, and then the call of the muezzin, calling the faithful to prayer. I turned to Graham and said, "You know, I'd forgotten this bit, isn't it wonderful!" and it was indeed.

The week went too quickly; I'd done little of what I wanted to do, I found that I didn't have the puff to snorkel or walk too far, without setting off the chest pain that was now getting worse. So home we came to a cold, wet, foggy UK.

A day later than planned, as we were delayed by technical problems, but naturally my first port of call was to see my GP and then the fun started with tests, scans at Papworth and Addenbrookes, all culminating in a verdict that I'd been incredibly lucky to get away with it, and now a different lifestyle was needed. With the treatment I was literally good as new, but had learned a sharp lesson that I was not as clever as I'd thought I was!

However, I'd still not completely finished with the Maldives. I'd been impressed with the amount of changes to the infrastructure, health care and so on for the locals, so I felt it worth commenting on that on my return. I wrote to the president saying as much, and to my surprise, within a fortnight received a reply from him, thanking me for my comments and wishing me and my loved ones all best wishes, and hoping that I would 'visit these shores again.' However, Pam's response to this was, "Not bloody likely!"

I treasure that letter – it's not everyone who has had best wishes from a head of state!

With so many memories and photographs, it would be difficult to forget the peace and tranquillity of the islands, and that will be with me until my dying day. I felt that I could truly say with the Psalmist 'I'd taken the wings of the morning and dwelt in the uttermost parts of the earth'.

So life proceeded apace, with few worries apart from support for my family when needed; they of course all suffered from the usual problems of life, but were a great source of comfort to Pam and I.

But then to upset the normal tenure of our way, my son Graham gave me a computer.

Given in kindness, but it caused me a lot of grief. I had little spare time to take a course in the art, so struggled on learning by my mistakes – not a good way to learn! – and now some ten years later still expect it to bite me, and it probably will!

My grandchildren of course are experts. What is wrong with grandparents I wonder? But I do object to being admonished by a robot when I've done some task incorrectly. It is an affront to my dignity when it goes dong! Technology and I are unhappy bedfellows. I'm sure I would have been happier in the steam age and Stephenson's Rocket. But then I would have probably regretted the passing of the stage coach and their horses!

Having been in practice for many years, I was now able to pick and choose those cases that were to me a greater intellectual challenge than the usual aches and pains I had seen in the past, but earned your bread and butter. The occasional case of alcohol addiction was always interesting to deal with. One patient said to me one day that he'd been to all the usual agencies for help but all they did was to preach at him. He told me that he knew what it was doing to his family and his liver, but wanted help, not censure. I asked him if he liked the taste of alcohol; he said he did. I told him that alcohol was a good friend but if treated badly, like all friends, it would become his enemy, and a couple of drinks a day would do him no harm in his circumstances. That cheered him up, as he contemplated a life without a drink with dismay, so by giving him a structured plan over the months, we ended up with having not a bottle-and-a-half of whisky a day, but two drams a day before bed!

Another patient I saw had a problem of 'not feeling well' but no physical illness was apparent or had been diagnosed. She lived in France; her husband worked for a UK defence company and was its European representative in that country where they had lived for the last four years. She didn't speak the language well, but was on holiday in Cambridge with friends who encouraged her to come and see me. It took a lot of unravelling, and some probing before the reason for the general malaise became apparent. Her self-esteem had taken a knock for some reason, but she was unwilling to open up. After a full physical examination as necessary had been completed, I asked about her habits and lifestyle. There was nothing out of the ordinary about these, but she felt she was letting everybody down and not fulfilling her desired role as wife and mother. She appeared full of remorse that in her husband's eyes and in that of the family, as she put it she was 'a waste of space'. I listened carefully to all this self deprecation with sadness. She really felt unworthy and unloved.

"You look tired," I said, "don't you sleep well?" She had dark rings under her eyes.

"Reasonably well," she replied, "but last night the thunderstorm was quite severe."

"You don't like storms?" I queried.

"It wasn't that, but my four-year-old daughter wanted to come into bed with me as she was frightened and wanted comforting."

"Into bed with you for comforting, why you? You are useless, you said so." The poor girl just looked at me, then her face crumbled and she burst into tears. I took both her hands in mine as I moved towards her.

Suddenly she said in a broken voice, "I'm not a murderer."

"I'm sure you're not," I said firmly, "do you want to tell me about it?" After a few moments it all came tumbling out. She'd had a lot of emotional and family pressure applied to encourage her to have a termination late in her pregnancy, for social reasons only she told me, and eight years later could still not forgive herself that the baby, who would have been a boy, was aborted at twenty weeks. In spite of the safeguards, always put in place by the clever people who wrote the act to stop unjust interference in a pregnant woman's life, there were even cleverer ones who knew how to get round them, and she had been coerced into an abortion. She desperately needed somebody to talk to who was independent and to comfort her in her ongoing distress. She had discussed having another baby after her two boys went to boarding school some ten years ago because she missed the boys so much, but her husband was against it, so as she told me, she stopped taking the pill. Her spouse was furious when he discovered her pregnancy. I spent a lot of time with her talking round the subject, and eventually with the help of a few needles she began to see the problem, and then I was able to get her to suggest ways of coping with it. I would never offer frank advice on this sort of problem, but by lifting the lid, as it were, on the problem as she saw it, I tried to guide her into finding an answer that was best for her, and that she could cope with.

Inevitably, those saddest cases I saw were of patients with terminal conditions. They knew I could do nothing to reverse their decline, but could I help them to cope with their problems?

There was a most useful organisation affiliated to the hospital called Hospital at Home. It was staffed by nurses and auxiliaries to support patients who had either been in hospital and had had surgery, and those who although still needing nursing care, needed to be kept an eye on so that their relatives could get a bit of peace to do the shopping and get some respite from their loved ones, so getting some relief from watching over them continually.

One day the nursing officer in charge of the organisation, an ex-patient of mine who knew my modus operandi, asked me if I was willing to see one of her patients, who following bowel surgery was finding it difficult to eat, because as soon as she took any of her diet she regurgitated it. She was losing weight of course and, as a young woman of forty, looked almost skeletal, which was most distressing to her husband, as he watched his once-beautiful wife turning into an aged wreck.

I visited her the same evening. She was a nice woman and desperately needed something to stop the spasm in her gastrointestinal tract. We talked about the problem for a while, then I examined her. I said, "Hmm, let's see what we can do."

She looked me straight in the eye and said, "Can I cry?"

I took her hand, "Of course you can, go ahead." And she sobbed for about five minutes. When she had simmered down I treated her for the vomiting, then stayed with her until she went to sleep. I went to find her husband and told him I would be back the following day, and next day after lunch went to see her. She was sitting up in bed drinking a cup of tea with an empty dinner plate in front of her. She looked at me and burst out laughing, "Look what I've done," she said, "enjoyed my lunch," and also she added, "I had a good breakfast after the best night's sleep I've had in weeks." To say that I was pleased was unnecessary but I said so anyway! She then said, "The doctor came this morning."

"What did he say?" I asked.

"Well I was eating my breakfast, he looked surprised and said that I looked better so the drugs were obviously working."

"And what did you say?"

"I told him I'd not taken any drugs, but an acupuncturist came to see me last night," she smiled impishly. "He just sniffed and made a face."

"And?" I prompted.

She looked cross. "I just took off," she said. "'He helped me,' I said, 'he let me cry, you told me not to, I wanted to hold your hand, and you took your hand away so I could not hold it and put my hand back under the sheet.'"

"Oh dear, stiff upper lip stuff, British eh?"

"Yes," she said, "but I'm not British, I'm Irish."

"So you are half emotion then," I observed and laughed with her. She lasted a few more months – her disease was malignant – but I like to think I helped along that dreadful road to her end. We all have to die; a good death should follow a good life, but sadly rarely does.

Geordie was another one who needed a friend. He had a wonderful wife whom he loved dearly. She was so distressed to see his terminal state, but like many people in love they kept their feelings from each other so as not to hurt each other. Oh dear, if only they realised how much better life would be if they bled emotionally over each other sometimes! However, he had come to see me with a severe lower backache. He had cancer of the gut and had already had massive invasive surgery. He was able to go back to work, his employers were most sympathetic and gave him a lighter job to do, but even that exhausted him. He was now fitted with an ileostomy bag which was most distasteful to him and added to his discomfort, and like so many people with such a bag he was embarrassed with the noise of his gut rumbling and the bag filling at inappropriate times, but after some six months the cancer had spread and very bravely he refused further treatment and as he put it to me, "I want to get it all over with, so it disturbs as few people as possible." He knew he was dying but soldiered on. He was a very gregarious man with a lot of friends, who he embarrassed by saying to them in the pub one evening when they were all together, "I hope you bastards will all come to my funeral and have all got decent suits, I don't want any scruffy sods there!"

There was little I could do for Geordie apart from massage his back and ease his pain slightly with heat and acupuncture, but I enjoyed seeing him and we had some quite hilarious sessions together. He had a fund of anecdotes and was an accomplished storyteller. He was a very courageous man, it must have cost him dear to be so cheerful, but one day when he came in he was looking old; I started with the usual queries and suddenly his voice broke and his face crumpled and the tears came. I just put my arms around him and gently massaged his back. We must have stood like this for half an hour, words were superfluous, and eventually he stood up, pulled on his shirt and said, "Thanks mate, you're a star," and walked to the door.

I knew I'd never see him again, "Goodbye Geordie," I said, "I'll be thinking of you," as he left the room.

Geordie died a week later, I was told, but some six months following his death I saw his wife in Tesco. She told me that he was at peace at the end, and also said that after he left me on his last appointment and arrived home in tears, he said to her, "Don was so bloody kind."

I would like to think that that phrase could be my epitaph.

So life continued, and Pam and I decided to improve our home before I finally retired; new carpets, curtains, furniture, new kitchen and so on. But of course, waiting in the wings was nemesis, and all our well-laid plans went into total tailspin.

Poor Pam became seriously ill with a dreadful malignant disease which required numerous hospital admissions, extensive surgery of the most horrendous kind and drugs by the ton, and all the paraphernalia of sickness took over our lives for the next two-and-a-half years.

Although after a few weeks it became apparent that this was not going to go away, I think we were both in denial until the end. The last week of her life, she was persuaded by her GP to go into the local hospice to have her drug regime assessed, he said. She agreed to go but only to give me a break, and after nearly three years I was pretty low. There is nothing so awful as to see the person you love most in your life disappearing before your eyes. She never complained, for three years she bore this dreadful disease with calm acceptance and very bravely. The most she ever said was that she was fed up with it all. The day came for her move to the hospice; she opened her eyes early morning after a fitful sleep, looked intently around the bedroom. I will never forget that look, I knew what she was thinking and said, "No darling, you will stay with me, you're not going anywhere."

With that she smiled at me, closed her eyes, never opened them again, and peacefully stopped breathing at 7.30 that evening with all the family round her.

I was completely gutted. I'd lost everything we'd worked for, I felt now as a comparatively young seventy-four year old I could only view the awful prospect of the future years without my dear girl. Why work, and for what?

But life did go on; I had so much help from my daughter Gillian and a couple of friends, both professional people, who were able to offer me their expertise, and some weeks after all the dust had settled, I took stock of what I had left and started to take an interest in work again. Also I had built up a body of knowledge from the experience, which now I could use to help others in the same boat.

One of the greatest problems however was going into an empty house at night, another coping with the embarrassment of those who knew me; they either avoided me when they saw me coming, or said the wrong thing when I met them, but this is a common problem with all newly-bereaved people. So, rather than imposing myself too much on my family, who were very busy people, I looked for another interest to fill the aching gaps in my day.

I was window shopping one afternoon and went past the local music shop. I glanced in the window and saw a row of keyboards on display. I stopped and thought, that's it, I could learn to play again!

I had been brought up with music. Both my brothers were musicians, my mother had a lovely soprano voice, and we spent many happy Sunday evenings around the piano singing our favourite hymns I had learnt to play the piano but had not touched an instrument for many years. The last time I had played was in 1964 when I was posted to Gan. There was a small Hammond organ in the chapel, I asked the padre permission to tinker on it, and eventually when the resident organist was posted home, the padre asked me if I would take over. I was a bit apprehensive, but had a stab at it, and eventually became the regular organist at evensong each Sunday. It certainly gave me a lot of pleasure; listening to music is one thing, but to make one's own is something else!

So I went into the shop and asked to hear some of these keyboard instruments. I was not impressed, and when the owner asked me about my experience in music I told him about playing the Hammond in Gan. He laughed, "Right," he said, "come with me." He took me over to a corner of the shop, and there was an organ identical to the one I'd played all those years ago! I had a go, found I could still play and bought it on the spot, to be delivered the next day.

When it was installed, it was such fun to make music again and it began to take up a lot of my leisure time. I even got up at night – it was fitted with headphones so I did not upset the neighbours – and as I became more proficient, I traded it in and bought a more advanced model, which was even more fun to use!

I was still working in the practice but really beginning to feel tired, and I was advised by my GP to get away from it all for a week. My brother and sister-in-law in Devon kindly invited me to spend some time with them. I had time to evaluate my life that week, and realised I could not go on at such a pace and would have to slow down or retire and go out on a high, or do something stupid due to tiredness, and have to pay the price.

As usual in my life, as one door closed, another opened, and it did this time again!

The Door Closes But Another Opens

It was then that I met Sandie again, who I had first treated in 1988 for her disability – she has MS. She had returned to Peterborough from Norfolk after the death of her husband. She had spent a lot of time in various homes and hospitals whilst living there, her husband was a very busy professional man which meant that he could not spend the time needed to care for her, but now that he had died she was completely on her own, being cared for by the social services; not a happy state of affairs, so she came back to be with the few friends she had in the city, and to start a new life here.

She phoned me and asked if I would treat her again. She had bought a small bungalow in a quiet part of the city, it had been adapted for her disability as she was now a paraplegic and was being cared for by the local authority care services.

We greeted each other as old friends, which we were; she'd been a lot of help to me when I was at the school of nursing and she acted as my model for practical teaching of nurses in the care of the young chronic sick. However, the friendship deepened in the months that followed. We were two very lonely people, and the inevitable happened; we fell in love, me at seventy-four, and she at 60! How this could have happened I still wonder all these years on; professionally it should not have happened, but it did!

One evening in late autumn I was sitting in my garden after a busy day in the surgery. It was very quiet, just the sound of distant traffic from the main road some way away and the birds singing. I relaxed thinking about things in general, when the first lines of a hymn I had last heard as a child came into my mind.

'Thy way, not mine oh Lord, however hard it be'. I went indoors, found my copy of good old hymns A and M, and read the rest of this poem. I went to bed that night still thinking about it and prayed for guidance; after all, my life was not easy on my own, as I had discovered, and I was very lonely.

I awoke next morning, and as I opened my eyes had the answer, and after breakfast went straight down to the bungalow, and in the time honoured tradition, on my knees, asked Sandie to marry me, and she did not refuse! So I closed the practice and was glad to.

We were married the following June on my seventy-fifth birthday, and so another wonderful chapter in my life began; what will this one bring, I wonder!

POSTSCRIPT

This has been the account of the third part of my life's journey; the second part I told in my previous book, *To Travel Hopefully*.

I am fortunate that by nature, I am and have always been an optimist, looking for another hill to climb, and by and large with a large dose of realism have achieved most things that I set out to do; but as the weeks and months pass by, I don't see any other major changes in my life, from now on. I am content now not to keep up the pace, unless I commit murder of my computer, which still gives me grief at times. I don't think that is a chargeable offence, but it would sometimes give me pleasure to see it confined to the dustbin!

Also, I have at all times been supported by my faith, ever-present when the need arose, and a vital component in my life whenever trouble struck. I think my attitude to religious belief has changed; I have come to see that telling me what I must do, ought to do, essential that I attend this or that ceremony, or say certain words at the appropriate time, I have come to see that it is not what a person does, but what he is that matters. It's not the man-made obligations created by persons and denominations who try to sell and own their brand of faith, with their own interpretations of what they think ancient texts mean, and hardly any of them agree with each other! And in times past would have willingly confined their opponents to the flames, and still would, had they the power to do so, but the basic understanding of what Our Lord taught us, and only that, to 'Love God and treat your neighbour as yourself' and 'In as much as you have done it to the least of one of these my brethren, you have done it unto me'. That surely is simple enough; in other words it's what you *are* that matters, not what you *have* to do, but what you should do, and if that simple commandment is adhered to, nobody would want or need to riot, be unkind, bully, lie, cheat or steal and so on; the list of evil is endless, and if they followed that principle, then the population of this Earth would start to live! And these same people with their sincere convictions will, along with myself when we arrive at the summit of our lives and pass from it, find within that 'better land' a lot of people who we thought could not by any stretch of the imaginations be citizens of that place and are awaiting us, but also a lot of others who we thought would be eligible for citizenship are conspicuous by their absence!

My life in alternative medicine has been completely satisfying, so different to that predicted for me by my nursing and medical colleagues, who all those years ago were unable or unwilling to see how anyone could possibly treat the sick without a full laboratory service, or X ray department, or drugs etc. These are vital things in the treatment of patients' illnesses. I know the benefits we have from modern medicine, but for a small number of patients there are ingredients missing in their care and treatment, and I think I was able to offer that in my practice, and the most important ingredients were time, kindness, attention and a listening ear.

Most of my successes have been with patients who have already trodden that road of medication without success. 'Here, take these tablets they will make you feel better', but they did not and found it to be a dead end, and I have been able to help them out of that cul-de-sac, and have vicarious pleasure in doing so for their own sakes. I shall always endeavour to think like this, but of course, Sandie comes first now, with all my energies going in her direction.

I have the satisfaction of knowing that the thorny path of my life has been so much more rewarding than I imagined it could possibly be when I set out on the journey all those many years ago. No, as St Paul said, 'Here we have no continuing city' – we are always moving on as we climb life's mountain to its summit.

The daughter of General Booth, the founder of the Salvation Army, in her later years whilst she was still working, was asked about her plans for the future. She said that she did not fear death, but didn't relish the idea of her demise were it to be caused by a painful condition, but averred that if the next world was anything like this one, and she believed it to be 1000 times better, what wonders awaited her when her time came!

So when my time comes and I truly arrive at the summit, I think I shall have the satisfaction of knowing that I have not wasted my life.

Sir Francis Drake is reputed to have said 'It is not the beginning, but the continuing of the matter until it be thoroughly finished which yields the greatest glory'.

I do not expect to go out in a blaze of glory, but when I arrive, hopefully somebody will be there to say 'Well done!'

THE END
(For the time being!)